Maria Kondratova

Cancer: Myths, Realities, and a Blueprint for Living

LiDER BOOKS

Kondratova Maria

Cancer: Myths, Realities, and a Blueprint for Living / M. Kondratova, 306 p.

Cancer is perhaps the most myth-riddled disease known to medicine. Many of these myths stem from actual scientific theories that have been twisted and distorted through years of retelling. In this book, molecular biologist Maria Kondratova of the Curie Institute in Paris cuts through the misconceptions to offer readers a clear, science-based understanding of cancer and current approaches to its diagnosis and treatment. Her work shows how molecular oncology has transformed our fundamental knowledge of genomics and cellular regulation into life-saving drugs and diagnostic tools. While cancer is undoubtedly a serious subject, this isn't just a book about illness and death. Rather, it's a testament to life itself—in all its complexity, vulnerability, and beauty.

Paperback: ISBN 978-965-93146-7-6
Hardcover: ISBN 978-965-93146-8-3
EPUB: ISBN 978-965-93146-9-0

Cancer: Myths, Realities, and a Blueprint for Living
Maria Kondratova

LIDER PUBLISHING LTD
Sheinkin 76, Givatayim
Israel
liderbooks.com

Managing Editor: Marina Krasavina
Project Editor: Natalia Pepelina
Translator: Sonja Swenson-Khalchenia
Copyeditor: Karen O'Donnell
Proofreaders: Beth Dymond, Katya Lutsky
Cover design: Yuri Buga

Paperback: ISBN 978–965–93146–7–6
Hardcover: ISBN 978–965–93146–8–3
EPUB: ISBN 978–965–93146–9–0

Table of contents

Preface

SCIENTISTS AND THEIR LOVE-HATE RELATIONSHIP WITH CANCER 11

COMMON MYTHS ABOUT CANCER 18

Chapter 1

MYTHS — BOTH HYSTERICAL AND HISTORICAL 21

HISTORICAL CONTEXT 23

ARE CANCER RATES RISING? 28

Maria Curie — an important name in the history of France as well as the history of cancer 32

BODY AND SOUL 34

THE TONGUE TALKS AT THE HEAD'S COST 36

DIAGNOSIS OR DEATH SENTENCE? 38

SUMMARY 41

Chapter 2

THE ENIGMA OF OUR GENOME AND MYTHS ABOUT THE NATURE OF CANCER 43

A GENETIC DISEASE 45

WHY DO CELLS NEED GENES? 48

THE GENETIC CODE IS BOTH DOGMA AND A ROADMAP! 55

THE GENOME STRUCTURE IS NO ACCIDENT 59

The world of RNA 65

HEREDITY AND VARIABILITY: WHY WE NEED MUTATIONS 68

CELLULAR DIVISION INEVITABLY LEADS TO GENETIC ERRORS 72

THE WIDE RANGE OF MUTAGENS 74

DOES EVERY MUTATION CAUSE CANCER? 80

BRCA — THE "ANGELINA JOLIE GENES" 84

IF YOU CANNOT BEAT THEM, TAKE CHARGE OF THEM! 88

SUMMARY 90
Chapter 3
CELL DIVISION SECRETS AND MYTHS ABOUT CHEMOTHERAPY 93
CHEMOTHERAPY – FOLLY OR NECESSITY? 94
CHEMO AND LIFE 97
CELL CYCLE OR LIFE CYCLE? 99
A VARIETY OF EFFECTIVE THERAPIES 104
Superheroes walk among us 107
WHERE SIGNAL PATHWAYS LEAD 109
TREATING THE SIGNALING PATHWAYS, BOTH INSIDE AND OUT 115
HUMANS AND DISEASE 119
SUMMARY 122
Chapter 4.
THE STORY OF HeLa AND MYTHS ABOUT DEATH AND IMMORTALITY 123
WHEN DEATH IS A BLESSING 125
APOPTOSIS – DYING TO LIVE 128
ONCOLOGY'S "STAR MOLECULE"–p53 133
TELOMERES – THE BODY'S BUILT-IN AGING SYSTEM 139
The story of HeLa 142
LIFE IN DEVELOPMENT 146
STEM CELLS – THE SOURCE OF ETERNAL YOUTH AND CANCER ALIKE 152
SUMMARY 155
Chapter 5
QUESTIONS ABOUT METABOLISM AND MYTHS ABOUT "EATING WELL" 157
THE SWEET FUEL OF LIFE 158
HOW THE WARBURG EFFECT ALLOWS US TO SEE THE TUMOR 162
SYMBIOSIS – THE ART OF SURVIVING TOGETHER 166

HOMEOSTASIS — WHY SIMPLE SOLUTIONS JUST DO NOT WORK 170
Mitochondria — the story of a single organelle 173
YOU ARE WHAT YOU EAT 176
GERMS ARE RIGHT AT HOME 179
MAGICAL THINKING AND SHARK CARTILAGE 184
SUMMARY 188
Chapter 6
THE TUMOR ENVIRONMENT AND MYTHS ABOUT METASTASES 189
CANCEROUS RUBICON 191
CANCEROUS TUMORS AS BOTH SUPERPARASITES AND "EFFECTIVE MANAGERS" 194
MYSTERIES OF THE BLOOD — ANGIOGENESIS 197
Seek, and ye shall find 200
OUR SECOND SKELETON 202
A WOUND THAT WILL NOT HEAL 207
FIND YOUR NICHE 211
SUMMARY 215
Chapter 7
THE FINER POINTS OF IDENTIFYING "THE OTHER" AND MYTHS ABOUT IMMUNITY 217
SPONTANEOUS REMISSION — A MIRACLE YOU CANNOT COUNT ON 219
GERMS AS CANCER FIGHTERS 221
TWO IMMUNE RESPONSES 223
KNOW THINE ENEMY 225
ANTIGENS AND ANTIBODIES 228
THE NATURAL ANTIGEN CYCLE 231
Allergies are a disease of clean hands 234
TUMORS AND IMMUNITY — AN EVOLUTIONARY DIALOGUE 236
THE IMMUNE RESPONSE FORMULA 241

BRINGING IMMUNITY BACK TO CANCER ... 243
WHY CANCER IMMUNOTHERAPY IS NOT INVINCIBLE (YET...?) ... 248
CANCER IS CONTAGIOUS BUT NOT IN HUMANS! ... 250
SUMMARY ... 252
Chapter 8.
A BRAVE NEW WORLD AND CONSPIRACY THEORIES IN ONCOLOGY ... 253
WHAT EVIDENCE IS THERE TO EVIDENCE-BASED MEDICINE? ... 255
A QUIET REVOLUTION — BIG DATA IN MOLECULAR ONCOLOGY ... 258
IN BOTH NUMBERS AND SKILL! ... 262
A doctor in your smartphone ... 265
THE CAT'S OUT OF THE BAG ... 267
PRECISION MEDICINE — A BRIGHT FUTURE AWAITS ... 275
Conclusion
MORE THAN JUST SCIENCE... ... 279
Afterword
PATHS TO SCIENTIFIC KNOWLEDGE — THE PARABLE OF THE BLIND MEN AND THE ELEPHANT ... 285
Acknowledgments ... 289
Bibliography ... 291
For the book in general ... 291
Chapter 1. MYTHS — BOTH HYSTERICAL AND HISTORICAL ... 291
Chapter 2. THE ENIGMA OF OUR GENOME AND MYTHS ABOUT THE NATURE OF CANCER ... 293
Chapter 3. CELL DIVISION SECRETS AND MYTHS ABOUT CHEMOTHERAPY ... 294
Chapter 4. THE STORY OF HeLa AND MYTHS ABOUT DEATH AND IMMORTALITY ... 295

Chapter 5. QUESTIONS ABOUT METABOLISM AND MYTHS ABOUT "EATING WELL" 297
Chapter 6. THE TUMOR ENVIRONMENT AND MYTHS ABOUT METASTASES 298
Chapter 7. THE FINER POINTS OF IDENTIFYING "THE OTHER" AND MYTHS ABOUT IMMUNITY 300
Chapter 8. A BRAVE NEW WORLD AND CONSPIRACY THEORIES IN ONCOLOGY 302
Afterword. MORE THAN JUST SCIENCE... 303
About the author: 306

Preface
SCIENTISTS AND THEIR LOVE–HATE RELATIONSHIP WITH CANCER

"When I want to read a novel, I write one." Most writers, including myself, would readily subscribe to this honed maxim of British statesman Benjamin Disraeli. After all, writers are first and foremost readers, and popular science authors are no exception.

For some time now, I have wanted to read (and therefore write) a book that is informative and also entertaining for a wide range of readers about the latest discoveries in biology, but the colossal task of what I wanted to do gave me pause. Where do you even start a project like that? Where should I focus? How could I draw connections between so many different, diverging facts into a single thread? And, finally, how could I convince non-biologist readers to dip their toes into one of the most interesting, complex areas of modern science, despite all of the inevitable difficulties for a layperson? I had no answers myself, and so I kept putting off actually writing the book.

As often happens, the question eventually answered itself. In 2014, I was offered a position at the Curie Institute, one of the world's leading molecular oncology research centers. Previously, I had never been particularly interested in cancer, and I only had a rudimentary grasp of the mechanisms of malignant tumors, mostly thanks to a medical biochemistry course I had taken two decades earlier. This made it all the more fascinating to open the door to a whole new field of knowledge. The deeper I delved into the subject, the clearer it became that cancer is not simply a disease, or even a group of diseases. Rather, it is a phenomenon that is as complex as life itself. It is even studied as living matter, at every level – from molecular to population (epidemiological) and even cultural levels. (Contemporary writer Susan Sontag, who died of leukemia, wrote many vivid, merciless pages about cancer in her philosophical work *Illness as Metaphor.*[1]) Cancer's impact on our lives goes far beyond the confines of medicine, making it not only a biological phenomenon, but also a cultural, social, and even political one. I became certain that cells' malignant transformation is much more than simply a disease after learning that cancer (like life!) is a phenomenon that has no definition.

Science begins with definitions: "An island is a piece of land surrounded by water," "Byzantium was a state founded following the division and breakdown of the Roman Empire," "Pushkin was a great Russian poet." The subject of biology – the science of living things – is not, in fact, strictly defined. Do not think for a second that scientists and philosophers have not been trying to answer the question "What is life?" all along. They have tried time and again, but each attempt somehow fails to do life justice and ends up feeling incomplete. After all, living things are inherently beyond being reduced to neat, unambiguous concepts. With good reason, they say that while physics and chemistry are the "sciences of rules," biology is the "science of exceptions." At the end of the day, in order to avoid wasting time on eternal debate, biologists decided to settle for rather loosely defined "signs of life," which are less a dogma than guidelines, and a very approximate boundary defining the "land of the living" from the material world.

---

1 Susan Sontag, Illness as Metaphor and AIDS and Its Metaphors. 1st ed. (New York: Picador, 2001).

Lists of these signs of life may vary from one textbook to the next but, in general, most authors agree that living matter is capable of maintaining a constant composition and internal environment (homeostasis), exchanges matter and energy with its environment (metabolism), and has a complex structure. Living things are capable of growing and reproducing. They react to changes in their environment and are able to adapt to external conditions. Finally (and I am adding this sign of life on my own behalf), once it has appeared, life, as a phenomenon, is able to exist and develop, apparently almost indefinitely, though the "immortality" of living things is generally achieved at the expense of its individual units — cells, organisms, species, and entire groups of living things, such as in the extinction of the dinosaurs.

Most strikingly, the majority of these features can be found at any level of existence of living things — from cellular to planetary (the biosphere). The most basic unit of life, the cell, has a complex internal structure, and the functions of its organelles generally replicate those of the actual organs in a multicellular organism. The ecosystem is capable of sustaining homeostasis. Following a forest fire, the forest is able to "heal its wounds" and recover, just as a damaged organ is able to recover its function in time. Individuals are capable of responding to environmental changes, but so are entire groups of animals and plants. The evolution of flowering plants is as impressive as that of the dinosaurs.

All of these basic features of life — the ability to grow and reproduce, sensitivity to environmental signals, a cellular structure — are found in cancer as well, albeit in a highly distorted, deviant way. Cell division, which is a necessary condition for any multicellular organism, becomes a cause of disease and death. The body's own ability to heal wounds begins to feed tumor growth. The way the body's own cells work together results in the immune system's inability to resist invasion. American physician and author Siddhartha Mukherjee writes about this feature of cancer in his book, *The Emperor of All Maladies:*

A Biography of Cancer:[2] "Confronting cancer is tantamount to confronting a parallel species, a species more adept at survival than ourselves."

For many years, scientists and doctors have attempted to find a more concise description of the essence of this disease, but they have consistently failed to do so. Two prominent oncologists, Douglas Hanahan and Robert Weinberg, suggested that colleagues take their lead from general biology and avoid any specific definitions, simply limiting themselves to listing cancer's "key features." Initially, there were six such features, then ten, and by the time this book has been finished and published, that number may have changed once again, but the point is the principle, rather than a specific figure. Each of these features is included in this book.

According to Hanahan and Weinberg, malignant tumors share the following features:

- genomic instability (Chapter 2)
- maintenance of cell division (Chapter 3)
- avoidance of growth-limiting mechanisms (Chapter 3)
- cellular immortality (Chapter 4)
- disruption of apoptosis (regulated cell death) processes (Chapter 4)
- energy metabolism disorders (Chapter 5)
- chronic inflammation (Chapter 6)
- invasion and metastasis (Chapter 6)
- increased vascular growth (Chapter 6)
- immune control avoidance (Chapter 7).

Some (and perhaps even most) of the items on this list may initially seem like inarticulate scientific jargon, but we will address each of them in this book.

---

[2] Siddhartha Mukherjee, Emperor of All Maladies: A Biography of Cancer. 1st ed. (New York: Scribner, 2011).

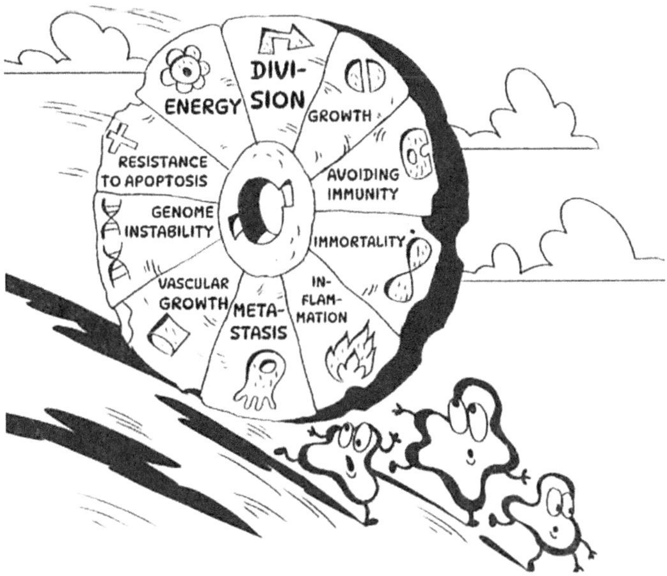

Figure 1. Not only do cancerous tumors differ from healthy tissues, but they are also very diverse among themselves. Within that diversity, however, they all share common key features that allow us to combine them into one disease group.

Why is it that cancer gets so much attention from researchers, whether they are physicians or biologists who study the most basic science, rather than focusing instead on scientific applications? When we observe the distortions inherent to malignant cells, scientists are better able to understand the molecular mechanisms in life's normal, healthy manifestations.

An early novel by brothers Arkady and Boris Strugatsky, *Noon: 22nd Century*, describes a humorous experiment by computer programmers working on a powerful supercomputer capable of creating material models of objects being studied. After teaching the computer to provide a normal description of a sheep, the mischievous scientists feed it an image of a five-legged animal with no cerebellum, and the poor computer begins to spit out monstrosities, trying to solve an unsolvable problem. When the cause of the anomaly is revealed, the programmers' colleagues first wanted to beat them in retaliation. However, the team then realizes that, thanks to the prank, their research group now has access to the largest collection of data on machine errors and is delighted with the new material for research and analysis.

If we look at cancer cells from the perspective of enthusiastic scientific curiosity, rather than superstition and horror, they are essentially the same five-legged anomalies, the victims of multiple errors — whether genetic, signaling, or metabolic in nature. However, by looking into this "warped mirror," we have a better understanding of life as it should be. Thanks to experiments on cancer cells, we have made numerous scientific discoveries, which I would like to describe in this book. You will see "Nobel Prize" mentioned at least ten times throughout the book, and not because I enthusiastically follow this prestigious scientific award, but because whether directly or indirectly, a significant portion of the past century's fundamental discoveries in medicine and biology have come from oncology research. As of the writing of this book, the 2018 Nobel Prize in Physiology or Medicine is the most recent example and was awarded for novel cancer immunotherapies based on immune response "checkpoints." Just as it was awarded, I was, in fact, making my final edits on that very chapter. There are many strange coincidences in life...

In the end, I did not write a popular science book about molecular biology in general, but specifically about cancer. I did not write about disease and death, but about life, and all of its complexities, perfections, and fragility. I am a researcher rather than a physician, and therefore it would be inappropriate for me to speculate about human suffering simply to grab readers' attention. For this reason, tragic "clinical" examples will be few and far between in this book, and in their place I have included detailed (and I hope optimistic enough) descriptions of molecular biology's successes. They say that basic science is "the satisfaction of personal curiosity at government expense." But any money taken from the state is taken from society as a whole, and any honest researcher should be ready to explain to people why certain resources should be spent on scientific developments rather than building a new stadium, roads, or social housing projects. Despite what scientists say, the connection between "good science" and a "good standard of living" is not always apparent to the average person. Molecular oncology is a rare and rather impressive example of how fundamental scientific knowledge about the genome's structure and cellular regulation systems has translated into drugs and diagnostic methods that have saved thousands of lives.

There are few diseases and few conditions of the human body (with the exception of perhaps pregnancy) that have been mythologized by our society as much as cancer. But when I began writing a book devoted to studying the most popular misconceptions in this field, my intention was not to act as a scientific prophet ridiculing and debunking others' ignorance. Myths, after all, are not born in a vacuum; they are a symptom that society — a wide range of laypeople — considers something to be an important issue, while lacking access to quality scientific information. As a result, people tend to try to answer these questions and fill these gaps with whatever they can. As we will see later on, many common myths about cancer are grounded in real scientific theories that have become distorted and mischaracterized with each retelling. This book aims to try to separate the wheat from the chaff while giving lay readers a simplified but accurate and, most importantly, scientific understanding of the nature of cancer and modern methods for its diagnosis and treatment. Myths belong in mythology, not medicine.

COMMON MYTHS ABOUT CANCER

All of us have heard one or more of the following "authoritative" statements on this list at least once:

1. A cancer diagnosis is a death sentence. No matter how you treat it, there is only one outcome.
2. Progress in cancer treatment? Don't be ridiculous. People were dying one hundred years ago, and they're still dying the same way today.
3. Before, there weren't such high cancer rates because people lived healthy lifestyles, in harmony with nature. And now, we have pollution, radiation, stress, cell phones... That's what causes cancer. It is a disease of progress, and there's nothing you can do about it.
4. Cancer is a hereditary disease, and if any of your close relatives have the disease, there's nothing you can do.
5. Cancer is a contagious disease. Have you heard of oncoviruses?
6. Cancer doesn't just happen. It's your own fault you got sick! You avoided cigarettes and alcohol, you exercised regularly, and you got it anyway? I don't believe it!
7. Cancer treatment is more dangerous than the disease itself. The tumor may still go away on its own, but chemo will definitely kill a person.
8. A cancerous tumor is capable of living forever, so cancer may hold the key to immortality.
9. A malignant tumor needs sugar; cancer is caused by having a sweet tooth!
10. Cancer "acidifies" the body, so on the contrary it must be "alkalized." Baking soda is a simple and effective cure for cancer.
11. Sharks don't get cancer, so shark cartilage is a proven means of preventing and treating the disease.
12. Metastases occur because the tumor has been "disturbed" by surgery or chemotherapy. If you leave it alone, it will not metastasize.
13. Cancer is an inflammation.

14. Folk remedies and immune boosters that strengthen the immune system can beat cancer. Have you heard of immunotherapy? That's what it is.
15. Folk medicine is as effective as modern medicine, and may even be better!
16. A universal cure for cancer was discovered long ago, but greedy pharmaceutical companies and corrupt doctors hide it from their patients in order to continue profiting from people's suffering.

We have counted sixteen such myths, but you may know more... In this book, we will take a close look at each of these common misconceptions and try to figure out what science really knows about each of the issues involved (the connection between heredity and cancer, the influence of lifestyle on the likelihood of suffering from the disease, etc.). We will take a frightening but fascinating journey through cancer as we try to understand the cellular mechanisms that turn healthy tissue into malignant tissue and learn how modern medicine is using the molecular features of cancer cells to develop new and effective means of diagnosing and treating the disease.

For readers who are interested, a full scientific bibliography can be found at the end of the book.

Chapter 1
MYTHS – BOTH HYSTERICAL AND HISTORICAL

Generally speaking, the myths surrounding cancer can be divided into two groups – optimistic myths offering a simple, universal explanation for its causes, along with promises of miraculous cures; and pessimistic myths, which twist our natural fear of disease into a state of hopelessness and despair.

It is hard to say which group does more harm. There are countless "optimistic" tales of people who managed to treat and cure their own disease, even at an advanced stage, while the pessimistic myths focusing on victims who suffer in silence get far less attention. But anyone who habitually avoids seeing a doctor (even when they are suffering from obvious and worrying symptoms) is playing deadly games with the toxic idea that "cancer is a death sentence – whether there is a cure or not, it all turns out the same way." It is difficult to quantify the number of victims of this kind of learned helplessness, but it is simply staggering.

Another popular and pessimistic myth is focused on the "good old days": "People did not get cancer in the past, but now, with pollution, stress, poor lifestyles..." This is a sort of new take on the legend of a "golden age," a mythical time of health, harmony, and prosperity, which was replaced by the ruthless "iron age" of modern civilization. This particular myth builds a general sense of doom, even among those of us who are perfectly healthy, and is a real obstacle to widespread methods for early detection and cancer prevention methods. After all, why bother taking vitamins and seeing the doctor if fate has it in for us all, anyway?

Is it true that people used to get cancer less often? Has there been any progress in treating cancer and diagnosing it, or is it still as deadly as it was fifty or a hundred years ago? Does psychological stress really increase your chances of getting sick in the first place? Before we dive into the cellular and molecular mechanisms of malignant transformations, we need to answer these burning questions.

HISTORICAL CONTEXT

A chronicle on the history of cancer is one of the best English-language resources devoted to the disease and opens by noting that "70–80 million years ago, there were cancer cells in dinosaur bones." With this one phrase, we can both start and finish the whole debate about the assertion that no one used to get cancer. Right in front of us, we can see that not even the dinosaurs could escape it. As for our hominid ancestors, the oldest fossils containing traces of cancer date back to 4.2–3.9 million years BC and belonged to upright humans (*Homo erectus*). Among mammals, humans are not alone when it comes to cancer. In fact, cancerous tumors are often found on human's best friends — cats and dogs. What is more, much of the scientific data contained in this book was obtained from laboratory animals — rats and mice that had developed neoplasms (tumors) that were often extremely similar to those that develop in humans. This similarity between humans and other mammals when it comes to cancer is what has made it possible to use animals to develop and carry out primary (preclinical) testing for new anti-cancer drugs.

There are descriptions of what appear to be malignant tumors and methods for treating them in medical documents stemming back to any ancient civilization — Egypt and Babylon, India, and China. In ancient Greece, Hippocrates studied cancer, and in ancient Rome, the great physicians Galen and Celsus did the same. The "father of medicine," Hippocrates, believed that the human body contained four humors, or fluids — blood, phlegm, and yellow and black bile — which he believed caused various diseases when they became imbalanced. According to this theory, cancer was caused by an accumulation of black bile. Ancient doctors observed that "melancholy fluid" was particularly prone to accumulating in the "loose" areas of the body, such as the "female womb" (uterus) and breasts. Based on these generalizations, breast and uterine cancers were already widespread, even in ancient Rome.

Ancient physicians treated cancerous tumors on the outside of the body with cauterizations and various ointments. Tumors on the inside of the body were simply not treated at all. Given the level of surgery at the time, this was the most humane and reasonable course of action. Of course, the tumor would kill the person eventually, but it did so relatively slowly, while any surgery in the absence of antiseptics and anesthetics would almost guarantee a quick, excruciating death.

During the seventeenth century in Europe, doctors viewed cancer as a parasite that devoured the patient's body. This concept became more widespread, and led to a new, unusual treatment method — pieces of raw meat were applied to the tumor. The idea was to give the patient some respite, as the parasite temporarily stopped eating away at their body and switched to what was offered instead.

For some time, cancer was seen as a contagious disease, just like the plague or leprosy, and cancer patients were isolated from society. Fortunately, this misbelief did not last very long.

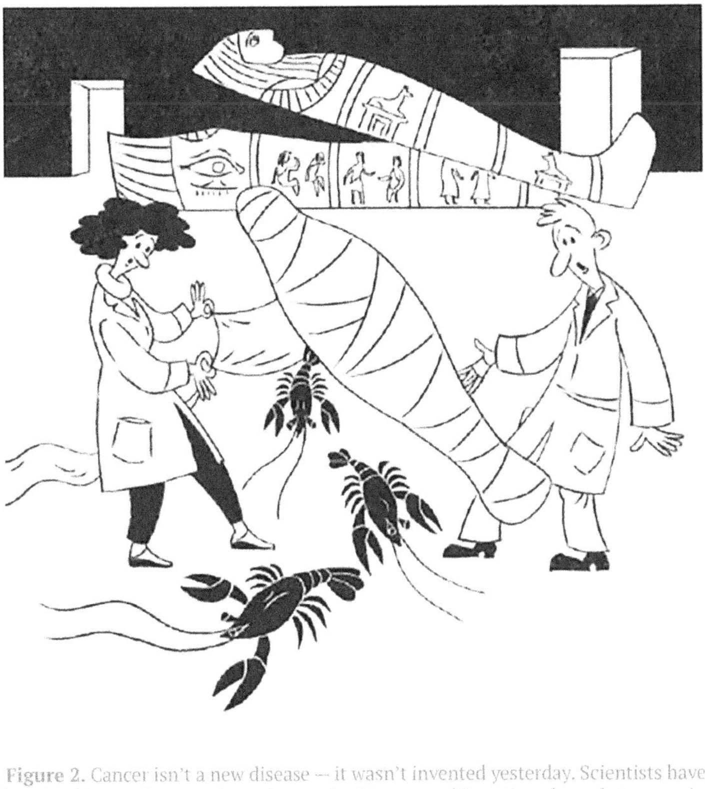

Figure 2. Cancer isn't a new disease — it wasn't invented yesterday. Scientists have found evidence of tumors in ancient animal bones and Egyptian pharaohs' mummies.

In the nineteenth century, for the first time, Johann Peter Müller and other prominent cytologists described cancer as a cellular pathology. Scientists demonstrated that metastases led to new tumors, which appeared as the result of the spread of malignant cells throughout the body. Around the same time, general anesthesia appeared, and medical surgery began to undergo rapid developments. Up until the early twentieth century, surgery was still the only cancer treatment available.

Unfortunately, however, removing the primary tumor did not necessarily mean that the patient would heal. The cancer would return, again and again. Surgeons began trying more radical methods, and in the late 1800s, when cutting out breast tumors, doctors began also removing the nearest lymph nodes, along with large chunks of the pectoral muscles, in order to prevent the cancer's return. Surgeries like this were a sure way to leave patients' bodies disabled, but, unfortunately, they did not guarantee a cure. The women who underwent these radical operations saw their tumors return almost as often as those who had less destructive procedures. There were also inoperable tumors and malignant blood diseases (leukemia), for which there were no surgeries available. By the dawn of the twentieth century, it was clearer than ever that our ability to treat cancer through surgery was limited by the very nature of the disease itself. Researchers began to search for ways to contain cancer cells' ability to multiply. Radiotherapy and chemotherapy thus appeared in oncologists' arsenal. This period also saw the first attempts to use the body's own defense mechanisms (Coley's toxins) against cancer, which we will discuss in Chapter 7.

The second breakthrough in diagnosing and treating cancer took place in the late twentieth century, when science took the next step deep into living matter: from cellular biology to molecular biology. We will discuss this "molecular revolution" in oncology in more detail below.

It is still too early to talk about our final victory over cancer, but since the 1970s, cancer survival rates have doubled on average, and in some cases those rates have now reached 80–95 percent. Unfortunately, not all tumors respond the same to therapy. Treating brain, pancreatic, liver, and lung tumors is still a challenge, even today. Early detection is the main factor when determining a patient's chances of recovery from any type of cancer. In their initial stages, most malignant tumors can be completely and permanently cured, but that likelihood drops dramatically as the tumor begins to grow and spread.

FACT: The term "carcinoma," or "crab-like tumor," was coined by ancient Greek physician Hippocrates, due to its external appearance, with outgrowths in different directions, which reminded scientists of a crab. The term was later translated into Latin by Roman scientist Celsus as cancer (crab), which then became part of international scientific language. In English, the fourth sign of the zodiac is known as Cancer, represented as a crab.

ARE CANCER RATES RISING?

"Sure, maybe cancer has always been around, but it was never this common before!" There is some truth behind this rather emotional statement, at least compared to the myth that people did not get cancer in the past. It is difficult to calculate how widespread cancer was in prehistoric times. In ancient burials, we usually only find bones, and not all tumors (even when they kill the person) leave traces of metastases in the hard tissue. Even data from the nineteenth century, which is not so long ago, has to be studied with caution. Most people did not have access to medical care, diagnostic tools were far from perfect, and medical statistics were not collected regularly.

But let us instead take a look at the last few decades. World Health Organization (WHO) statistics confirm that cancer rates are indeed rising. In 2008, 7.6 million people around the world died of cancer. In 2015, that figure had reached 8.8 million, and by 2030, if the trend continues, 13 million people per year will die of cancer. Clearly, cancer rates are on the rise — but is that bad news?

Even asking that question seems blasphemous. What can possibly be worse than cancer?! But just wait a moment before you get angry with me. While it is true that anyone can get cancer, medical statistics convincingly show us that it is first and foremost a disease of the elderly. (There is, however, a small group of pediatric cancers that primarily affect children under the age of five.) Young and middle-aged people are far less likely to get cancer.

In traditional societies, with very high child and infant mortality rates and early deaths among the elderly, cancer was not much of a problem. Today, about two-thirds of cancer patients in the United States are over the age of sixty-five, and this group has the highest cancer death rate. A hundred years ago, not as many people lived to be this age. Today, there is a clear trend toward higher cancer death rates in developed countries, rather than in developing countries. Does this mean that people in Africa or Latin America are healthier? No, but on average they have much shorter lifespans, and their causes of death tend to be dominated by other factors — hunger, infectious diseases, and injuries, for example. Moreover, many cancers are simply not diagnosed. Just as in nineteenth century novels, many fatal diagnoses were reduced to a brief period of withering away. Today, in many regions of the world, poor people still die of unspecified causes. A person lived and died, but from what? Only God knows... Therefore, it is a fallacy to claim that modern society gave us cancer. A much more accurate statement would be that "modern civilization's advancements allow us to live long enough to get cancer."

Of course, it would be too optimistic to claim that rising cancer rates are only due to enjoying longer lifespans. Industrial pollution and bad habits, especially smoking, also contribute to cancer rates. However, we need to be critical of today's challenges and take steps to fix them, rather than idealizing the past. Living in harmony with nature, as we imagine it today — working in the open air; eating a rich, diverse diet; sleeping well; having healthy sexual relations — was a rare, expensive privilege that was historically only available to very few members of the human race. The vast majority of our ancestors lived and survived quite differently.

One common disease among London's lower classes during the seventeenth to nineteenth centuries was known as soot wart, or "chimney sweep's carcinoma." This was a malignant testicular tumor that frequently developed among young men who as children (from ages five to twelve) had worked as chimney sweep assistants — their job was to climb into chimneys and clean them from the inside. Soot from the chimneys would eat its way into the boys' bodies, including through the delicate skin of the scrotum, and ten to fifteen years later, they would develop a tumor. In 1788, English doctor Percivall Pott, who studied this pattern, succeeded in convincing parliament to ban the employment of children under the age of eight as chimney sweeps. Unfortunately, the law was ineffective — employers were happy to simply pay the fines and continue exploiting young children. Pott's grandson, Henry Earle, continued his grandfather's research and found new evidence linking child labor exploitation and this dangerous disease. By the mid-nineteenth century, the laws were finally tightened, and no one under the age of twenty-one was allowed to work as a chimney sweep. However, these strict measures still did not have the desired effect.

Even the invention of a new chimney-cleaning machine did not manage to seriously make a dent in the situation. Insurance companies continued insisting on using boys as chimney cleaners, as they felt that the machines did not clean as well as the children did. The story dragged on for another century, and soot wart was not completely eradicated until the twentieth century, when apartment buildings stopped using fireplace heating altogether. Of course, today, we have many more dangerous substances to deal with than one hundred to two hundred years ago, but we are also much more careful around them than our ancestors were. It is impossible to imagine a story like the one described above happening in modern England. In this book, we will examine cancer through the prism of discoveries in molecular biology. This is, of course, fascinating, but there are certain distortions. Most horrible diseases of the past were defeated less by groundbreaking scientific discoveries (such as the invention of antibiotics) than by methodical, boring preventive measures carried out consistently over a lifetime.

Monitoring drinking water and food quality, providing preventive vaccinations, and quarantine measures all help prevent the development of epidemics. Along with promoting a healthy lifestyle, these represent the major achievements of public healthcare in developed countries. We are inspired by the day-to-day battles waged by doctors, but a truly effective health policy is less focused on treatment and more on prevention. Since the second half of the twentieth century, this approach, which has shown its effectiveness in the face of many infectious diseases, was finally applied to cancer as well. Monitoring industrial pollution levels, anti-smoking campaigns, and widespread advertising of the benefits of sunscreen are measures that save more people from cancer each year than all of the molecular biology achievements that we will be discussing in this book. Slowly but surely, this approach to safety is paying off. In developed countries, over the last several years, there has been a marked decrease not only in cancer-related deaths, but also in the numbers of new cases. The road ahead is still long. Experts believe that at least 30 percent of cancers could have been prevented by avoiding unhealthy habits and taking advantage of available preventive measures.

FACT: According to the National Cancer Institute (US), the likelihood of getting cancer for humans is highest between the ages of fifty-five and seventy-five. After the age of seventy-five, it begins to drop, and by eighty-five it is almost as low as among younger age groups.

Maria Curie – an important name in the history of France as well as the history of cancer

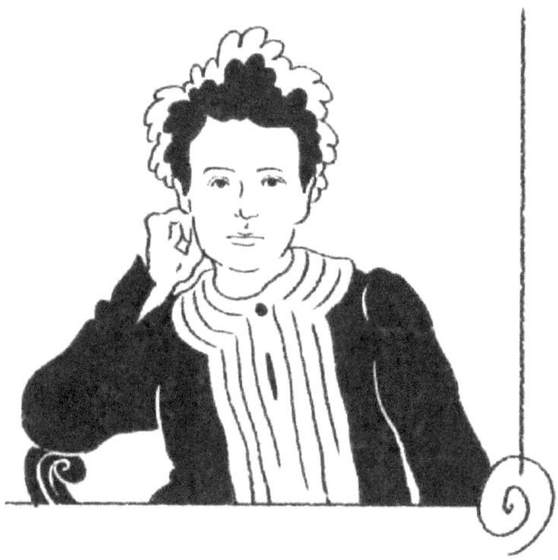

Marie Curie (née Maria Skłodowska) is renowned for her role in the discovery of radium and the study of radioactivity, but in France she is also revered as one of the founders of cancer research. In 1909 (six years after receiving the Nobel Prize for the discovery of radium, and three years after her husband Pierre Curie was killed by a horse-drawn carriage), the University of Paris and the Pasteur Institute decided to build a new research center – the Radium Institute.

Marie Curie was asked to lead it. The new research organization was dedicated to the study of potential applications of radioactivity in physics, chemistry, biology, and medicine. Marie Curie led the physics division, while Dr. Claude Regaux was in charge of the biology and medical divisions. Together, they founded radiotherapy, a method for treating cancerous tumors with doses of radiation. (Interestingly, it was Pierre Curie who had first suggested medical applications of radiation in fighting cancer shortly before his death.)

The Radium Institute quickly began to make advancements and grow. By the 1920s, with financial support from Henry Rothschild, it began working alongside the Curie Foundation. In 1970, these two organizations were merged, forming the Curie Institute, an independent research and medical center. Today, the Curie Institute (which has several branches in addition to the central Paris office) employs over three thousand people around the globe, and its hospital treats thousands of patients each year. The center's main areas of scientific and applied research are breast cancer and pediatric oncology (cancers in young children, such as retinoblastomas). The first floor of the former Radium Institute is now home to the Curie Museum, which is dedicated to the history of the discovery of radioactivity. Nearly a hundred years after her death, the story of Marie Curie, a conscientious girl from Warsaw who spent years working as a governess in order to pay for her own education, is an inspiration for young women everywhere who have decided to devote their lives to science, whether physics, chemistry, or biology.

From the windows of the top floor of the Curie Institute, you can see the edge of the Panthéon dome, the final resting place for many famous people in French history — writers, politicians, artists, and scientists. The ashes of Pierre and Marie Curie have also been there since 1995, after they were solemnly transferred from a modest cemetery in the Parisian suburb of Sceaux.

BODY AND SOUL

This book deals primarily with the biology of malignant tumors, but humans are biologically very special. We have the gift of reason, will, and the ability to experience complex, sometimes contradictory feelings. Despite all of the advances described above, cancer is undoubtedly a serious disease, which affects both body and soul. This is likely why, when it comes to cancer, questions about the link between the "spiritual" and the "physical" are so troubling to us all, whether we are healthy or sick.

We all go through difficult periods in our lives — the death of a loved one, divorce, illnesses, losing a job. No one is immune to psychological stress. How do negative feelings influence our cancer risk?

Here is some good news — as of today, there is absolutely no reliable evidence that psychological distress has a direct influence on whether or not we develop a malignant tumor. This means that the link between stress and heightened cancer risk is either nonexistent or too weak to be detected by standard statistical methods. Even suffering from long-term mental anguish, as is the case in those with depression, does not appear to increase your cancer risk, according to numerous data sets. If you are going through a rough period in life, there is no need to add worrying about cancer to your troubles.

However, that does not mean that life's challenges do not indirectly contribute to cancer. Often, people attempt to deal with stress by smoking or abusing alcohol, or generally not taking care of their health. Stress itself may not cause cancer, but bad habits certainly do. And though we cannot always control or prevent psychological distress, we can control our own self-destructive coping mechanisms.

A cancer diagnosis itself is a major stressor, and there is no doubt that a patient's ability to manage that can have an impact on their chances of recovery. Experiments on mice have shown that when subjected to social isolation (a form of stress), the animals experience accelerated tumor growth and metastases. This may be related to the fact that stress hormones, such as noradrenaline, can affect tumor cell metastasis and the immune system, which, as we will see later on, plays an important role in inhibiting tumor growth.

There is therefore good reason to believe that emotions such as despair, helplessness, and hopelessness increase the risk of a premature death, even without a cancer diagnosis (though the mechanisms of this phenomenon are still unclear). This means that patients should be provided with psychotherapy and, in some cases, with antidepressants chosen by their physician. Major cancer centers often have psychologists who specialize in cancer patients and are available for both patients and their loved ones. This is an important aspect of treatment that should not be neglected.

Though timely psychological and spiritual support is important to anyone in distress, including someone with a cancer diagnosis, we should not exaggerate its impact on the patient's outcome. Nothing compares to an early diagnosis and appropriate treatment when it comes to successful recovery. Mind power alone cannot cure cancer, no matter how much some may try to insist on it.

> **FACT:** Contrary to popular belief, in most religious traditions, including Christianity, spiritual practices (prayer, meditation, taking part in religious rites) are in no way in conflict with going to the doctor. The Old Testament directly speaks about the fact that medicine pleases God: "Honour a physician with the honour due unto him for the uses which ye may have of him: for the Lord hath created him" (Ecclesiasticus 38:1). Refusing medical care for a serious illness in hopes that one's "spiritual strength" will be enough is nothing short of arrogance. In other words, "Trust in God, but do not make things worse for yourself."

THE TONGUE TALKS AT THE HEAD'S COST

Many misconceptions about cancer are rooted in the inaccuracies and conservatism of language itself, which has not kept up with scientific discoveries. Even the way we talk about "breast cancer" and "colon cancer" gives the impression that we are talking about the same disease that just happens to be affecting different organs. For example, we might talk about "pimples on your arm" or "pimples on your back," though from a dermatologist's point of view, these are not the same types of pimples at all. When we talk about someone having a "rash," that may be a symptom of various issues, and it will be treated based on what caused it. An allergic rash is treated differently from juvenile acne, and chickenpox is treated differently from scabies.

This is also the case for malignant tumors. Cancer is not a monolithic disease, but a whole group of diseases with a number of shared symptoms, the most important of which are rapid, uncontrolled growth of the neoplasm and spreading throughout the body (metastasis). There are now at least four molecular subtypes of breast cancer alone. This detailed classification is not just a way for bored specialists to keep themselves busy. The tumor's molecular type will determine which drugs and therapies will be most effective in treating the disease, and what works for one type may be contraindicated for another. Another example of this is lung cancer. The term itself encompasses at least four types of disease: small cell cancer and non–small cell cancer, which itself is divided into three more types: adenocarcinoma, squamous cell carcinoma, and large cell carcinoma, each of which requires its own specialized treatment.

Classifying cancers is further complicated by the fact that the specific molecular tumor type (e.g., "luminal subtype A breast cancer") might have several stages — a localized tumor, a tumor that has metastasized to adjacent lymph nodes, and a tumor that has metastasized and produced secondary tumors in distant organs. Treatment methods and chances of recovery also differ between each of these stages.

This is not to say that generalizations like "cancerous tumor" are pointless. Malignant neoplasms of very different origins share many features (at both the cellular and the molecular levels), which define general cancer treatment strategies. These similarities are reflected by the way we talk about them and the general term "cancer" that is used to describe them, but that means that we have to keep in mind that differences do exist.

In this book, in a concession to natural language, I will use the terms "malignant tumor (neoplasm)" and "cancerous tumor" as synonyms. Strictly speaking, however, this is not entirely correct. Originally, the definition of "cancer" referred only to carcinomas — tumors formed by a specific type of cell, that is, epithelial cells. Tumors formed by connective tissue would be correctly referred to as "sarcomas," or the malignant deterioration of hematopoietic tissues as "lymphomas" and "leukemias," etc. However, in English, the term "cancer" has for some time now been used to describe all malignant diseases (which we can see when reading the monograph of the same name by the great oncologist Robert Weinberg). The term "tumor" will by default imply a malignant tumor, without any qualifying adjectives.

Throughout the book, these terms will be used when discussing the common features shared by various malignant neoplasms. When describing the characteristics of a specific type of tumor, I give preference to more precise terminology: "Ewing's sarcoma," "melanoma," "stomach cancer," etc.

FACT: Cancer is not one single disease, but a whole group of diseases.

DIAGNOSIS OR DEATH SENTENCE?

In order to understand whether fears of a "cancer sentence" are well founded or not, we will need to look at medical statistics. However, we also need to be careful and consider the context when looking at cold, hard numbers, keeping in mind the well-known joke that taking temperatures in the morgue and the infection unit (where patients often have a temperature of over 40 °C/104°F) simultaneously will give the hospital's patients an average temperature of 36.6 °C (98.6°F), indicating that they must all be in perfect health.

At first glance, cancer statistics seem to confirm our worst fears. The main criterion for successful cancer treatment is a patient's five-year survival rate after diagnosis.

In Russia, that rate is about 40 percent, which is unfortunately about the same as survival rates based on American data from the 1970s. In Western Europe and the United States, things are looking more optimistic, at 60–70 percent. Contrary to popular belief, cancer treatment in major Russian cities does meet global standards. So, what can possibly explain the nearly twofold difference?

The main factor in determining a patient's survival odds is the stage at which the cancer is detected. To give you one example, here are some treatment statistics from the United States for the most common type of "female" cancer, breast cancer. For a tumor found in the early stages, the chances of survival five years after diagnosis are close to 100 percent, but for a tumor diagnosed at stage four (with multiple metastases throughout the body), that figure is only about 20 percent. (The five-year survival criterion is used in oncology because it is during the early years that the cancer is most likely to recur. If malignancy has not returned within five years, it is highly likely to have been permanently cured, though later recurrences do unfortunately happen.)

In Russia, the main problem with cancer treatment continues to be late diagnosis. Regular examination by specialists does not require significant financial expense, and it can greatly increase one's odds of beating the disease. Of course, it is not possible or practical to be tested for every possible type of tumor each year, but a timely diagnosis is possible for nearly all of the most common types of cancer.

According to the WHO, the most common types of cancer for men are lung, liver, stomach, colon (colorectal and rectal), and prostate cancers. For women, they are breast, lung, colon (colorectal and rectal), cervical, and stomach cancers. Regular (annual) screenings of these organs ensures that if cancer occurs, it will be treated.

Vaccination against hepatitis B and preventing hepatitis C dramatically reduces one's chances of getting liver cancer. Quitting smoking minimizes the risk of lung cancer and reduces the risk of many other cancers. Regular gynecological exams can detect cervical cancer and early-stage breast tumors, etc. These and other preventive measures, which we will discuss further in detail, are available to most people and do not require a significant financial investment, with the exception of colonoscopies and gastroscopies to diagnose colon and stomach tumors, though these can be performed every few years.

Why is it, then, that despite obvious advancements in the field of oncology, people continue to believe in fatalistic myths and avoid doctors, preferring to put their health in the hands of charlatans? Naturally, there are many reasons for this, but the most important appears to be the idea of a "survivor error" in statistics whenever there is a lot of data on one group (survivors) and little on the other (those who died). This results in a skewed view of the situation. The name of this fallacy likely goes back to the story of the ancient Greek sage Diagoras of Melos, whose friend was trying to persuade him to believe in the existence of gods by showing him images of people who had survived a storm because they prayed to immortal intercessors. Diagoras of Melos very elegantly responded by asking, "What about the images of those who prayed, but died anyway?"

We can compare this story to the informational bias when it comes to cancer. Only in cancer cases is it more appropriate to speak of "death error" rather than "survivor error." There are many well-known stories of famous people who died of cancer: Steve Jobs, Chadwick Boseman, Patrick Swayze... People think, "If all of their intelligence, talent, influence, and wealth did not save them, what hope do the rest of us have?" as they read through news feeds and obituaries. Stories of people who have actually beat cancer are much less widespread in the news. Generally, no one other than those closest to a person know they have been diagnosed with cancer. If a person dies, then people may discuss the cause of death at the funeral. But if they recover, the illness will remain a mystery to others. This leads to very one-sided information, and an overly pessimistic picture. Meanwhile, around the world, there are tens if not hundreds of millions of people who have successfully beat cancer (there are over twelve million in the United States alone). Today, a cancer diagnosis is certainly an ordeal and a challenge, but it is in no way a death sentence.

FACT: Hollywood actor Robert De Niro was diagnosed with cancer in 2003. Eighteen years later, he is still with us. In the 1990s, stock trader Nassim Taleb was diagnosed with laryngeal cancer. Ten years later, his book, The Black Swan, became a bestseller, and by 2018, he was recognized as one of the world's most influential intellectuals. There are many more such stories with happy endings than we realize.

SUMMARY

Cancer has been a part of human life for centuries. Descriptions of cancerous tumors and treatment methods can be found in the medical annals of all ancient civilizations, though cancer did not become a serious epidemiological problem until the twentieth century. This can partly be explained by the spread of bad habits (smoking, excessive time in the sun), and partly due to the influence of industrial pollution. The main factor, however, is simply the increase in life expectancy that we have seen over the last several decades.

It is important to remember and understand that "cancer" is not simply one disease (as is the case with influenza or tuberculosis), but an entire group of diseases with different causes, albeit with similar external features. In this chapter, we have discussed several social and psychological aspects of cancer, and in the next, we will begin to analyze the molecular nature of this cellular pathology.

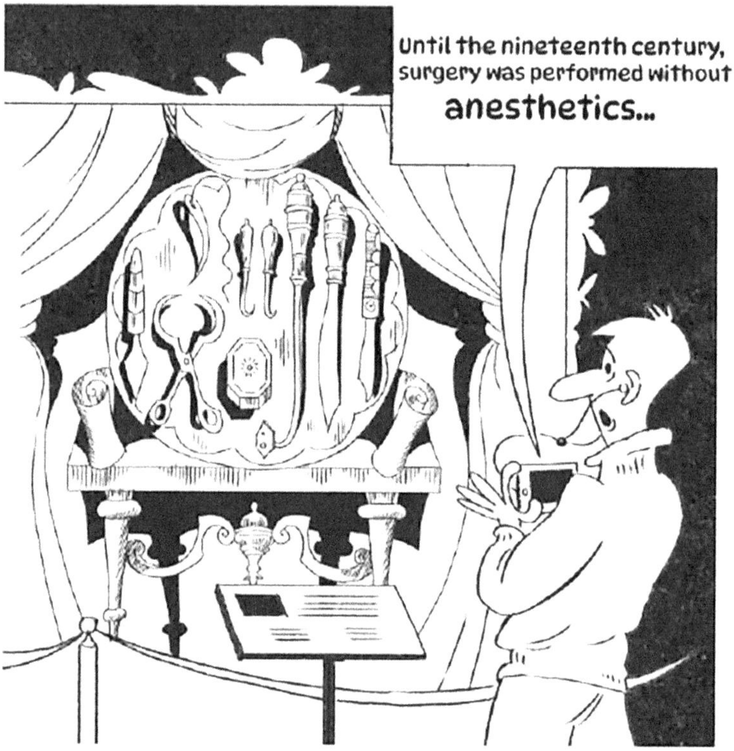

Figure 3. Surgery continues to be a very important cancer treatment, but many other methods have been added over the past one hundred years.

Chapter 2
THE ENIGMA OF OUR GENOME AND MYTHS ABOUT THE NATURE OF CANCER

The next group of misconceptions about cancer can be characterized as myths about its nature, which tend to be a whimsical amalgamation of scientific facts and collective speculations. Any ordinary layperson who attempts to delve into the origins of cancerous tumors will understandably feel confused with so many concepts that, at least initially, appear to be almost random. We know that at least some of our genes play a role in whether or not we get cancer, and that doctors often ask about cancer in our families. Does that mean that cancer is a genetic disease? At the same time, however, oncology literature often talks about oncoviruses — does this mean that cancer is a viral infection? And if so, does that mean it is contagious? Then again, if we read publications for the general public that talk about carcinogens, we come away with the impression that cancer is a type of "poisoning"... What causes cancerous tumors is not an easy question to answer. Cancer is complicated and involves many different factors. In this chapter, we will attempt to outline modern scientific understanding of its nature.

"Cancer doesn't just happen; it's your own fault you got sick!" This is something that many people hear after being diagnosed with cancer. Yes, it is hard to deny smokers' responsibility for the development of lung cancer but, often, people who lead perfectly healthy lifestyles get sick too. Understanding the mechanisms of malignant cell transformation can free patients and their loved ones from unbearable and unproductive feelings of guilt, and remind healthy people that, unfortunately, there is no way to guarantee they will not get sick themselves.

A GENETIC DISEASE

In 1928, English doctor Frederick Griffith conducted an experiment in which he injected healthy laboratory mice with a mix of two varieties — rough and smooth — of the bacteria that causes pneumonia. Based on earlier experiments, he already knew that only smooth forms of pneumococcus are dangerous to animals, as the microbial cell is surrounded by a capsule, which protects the bacteria from being recognized and destroyed by the mouse's immune system. The rough bacteria do not have such protection, and a healthy animal's body can easily fight them off, so that the animal does not get sick. Whether or not the bacteria have a shell was a genetic feature passed on from one generation to the next.

In an experiment that would later be described in biology textbooks, the smooth bacteria were killed with heat and then added to live rough bacteria. Individually, neither the killed smooth pneumococcus nor the live rough variety had any effect on the health of the mice. However, after they were injected with a mix of live rough and killed smooth bacteria, they developed pneumonia.

At the same time, live smooth bacteria were detected in the blood of the sick mice. Based on these observations, Griffith concluded that there was some component of the killed smooth cells that was transforming the rough bacteria (which did not cause disease) into smooth bacteria (which did). This was the first demonstration that heredity has a material nature and a material carrier that is capable of retaining features (at least for a while) even after the death of an organism.

In 1944, laboratory methods had improved, and some other researchers — Avery, MacLeod, and McCarty — conducted a similar experiment, in which they were able to isolate the mysterious "transforming agent" and describe its chemical nature.

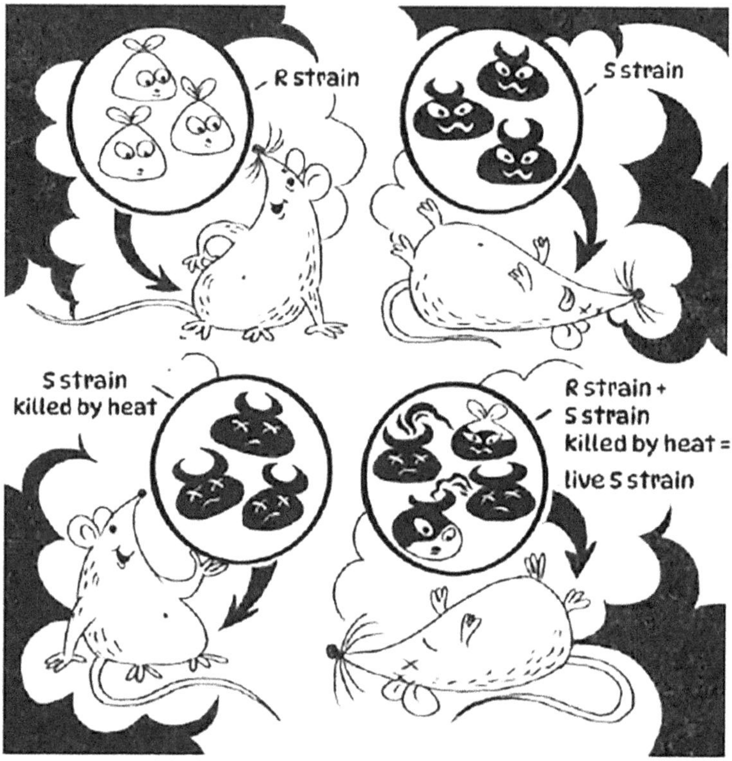

Figure 4. In Griffith's experiment, non-aggressive bacteria (R) captured DNA fragments from the killed bacteria (S). As a result, R bacteria changed (transformed)—they acquired the ability to synthesize a protective capsule and become dangerous to mice.

Deoxyribonucleic acid (DNA) molecules turned out to be the carriers of genetic information, and a new science — molecular biology — was born.

Since that time, terms like "genetic code," "mutation," and "heredity" have become household terms and frequently even appear in the tabloids (perhaps the highest form of popularity and acceptance).

Though only a small number of specialists truly have a detailed understanding of the complex molecular machinery underpinning life, the general idea that each organism has a unique DNA sequence (genome) is now part of general scientific culture and knowledge, just like "the earth rotates around the sun," "plants give off oxygen," and "it all started with the Big Bang." Since its inception, the main goal of molecular biology has been to explain the links between an organism's DNA sequence and its biological properties — or, as researchers themselves like to describe it, between the genotype (for example, the gene for green eyes) and the phenotype (actually having green eyes). Biologists have made impressive strides in this area, though there is a long way to go before we have fully deciphered the fundamental "code of life." On the contrary, the old parable of philosopher Anaximenes rings truer than ever — the more we expand our circle of knowledge, the more we realize our own ignorance, and the more questions we have.

In 1981, over fifty years after Griffith, researchers repeated his experiment, but using a malignant tumor rather than bacteria. They carefully extracted DNA from the tumor cells and transferred it to healthy cells in mice, after which they turned (transformed) into cancer cells. Thus, the genetic nature of cancer was discovered — not that anyone had any doubts about it. Over time, the link between genes and disease had long since been established, but actual direct evidence was needed in order to move forward.

While molecular biology attempts to understand the structure of healthy cells, molecular oncology is interested in how disorders in certain genes can lead to malignant transformation, and how we can correct them.

FACT: Cancer cells differ from normal cells within the same genome.

WHY DO CELLS NEED GENES?

If sociological surveys are to be believed, many people are still convinced that genes only exist in genetically modified organisms and food, and that they are absent in "normal" ones... This is why, before delving into the exciting topic of genetic disorders in tumors, we should take a look at how a live cell in a human body is structured, and why it needs genes.

A cell is the basic unit of living material (let us leave arguments about viruses to the experts). As the minimum "atom of life," it has all the signs of living material, to a greater or lesser extent — it grows, multiplies (divides), exchanges substances and energy with its environment, and adapts to changes in that environment. There are two main types of cells: "non-nuclear" (prokaryotic), for example, bacteria; and "nuclear" (eukaryotic), some unicellular and all multicellular organisms. When talking about cancer, we will be mostly interested in the second type — eukaryotic cells.

A unicellular organism is similar to a simple, rural household in the Middle Ages, which provided itself with everything it needed — from clothes and shoes to food, only exchanging things with the outside when absolutely necessary. (For example, peasants would sell some of their crops in city markets and use the proceeds to buy iron tools they needed from the blacksmith.) A multicellular organism is more like a modern, industrial city. In a megalopolis, each resident has their own specialty: a bus driver might not know how to bake bread, and a doctor might only have a vague grasp of advancements in modern astronomy. Cells also have different occupations, and just like in human society, the process by which they acquire these skills is called "specialization," or "differentiation." In the human body, there are about two hundred different types of cells, and each one has its own function — red blood cells carry oxygen, liver cells filter hazardous substances, neurons transmit electrical impulses.

Cells of the same type work together, like factory workers, forming tissues, such as nerves, muscles, skin, etc. These tissues, in turn, form organs which are specialized to perform specific functions — for example, lungs are for breathing, the stomach is for digestion. The structural hierarchy of the human body is body — organs — tissues — cells.

Living begins with the separation of "me" and "not me"—cells are separated by a thin membrane that makes it possible to not dissolve into their environment, thus carrying out a protective, insulating function, while also transporting necessary substances. This is a cell membrane property known as selective permeability. The membrane is composed of lipids (fats) and proteins. Lipids are responsible for insulation, while proteins transfer substances (this is performed by transport proteins), and cells react to signals from the outside world (this is the function of receptor proteins). Inside the membrane, there is a dense, concentrated solution known as the cytoplasm, which makes up the inner cell environment.

In a bacterial cell, DNA floats in the cytoplasm, but in nuclear organisms, such as human beings, hereditary information is stored in a special cellular component called the nucleus. At first glance, this may not seem like a major difference but, biologically, it is highly significant. In bacteria, all stages of implementing biological information take place simultaneously. Messenger ribonucleic acid (RNA) is read from the active gene, and ribosomes immediately sit on it, ready to synthesize the necessary proteins. In the cells of nuclear organisms, these two processes (reading and writing the genetic code) are divided by both time and space. RNA is read in the nucleus, while it is written (the protein is synthesized) in the cytoplasm. This slows the process down to a degree, but also makes it much easier to control.

"Control" or "regulation" are two key words that you will see time and again throughout this book. Eukaryotic (nuclear) and prokaryotic (non-nuclear) cells use the same molecular mechanisms, more or less, though only nuclear cells are capable of forming a multicellular organism. The key factor behind this evolutionary success is likely to be these cells' ability to more precisely regulate the molecular processes going on around them.

The existence of a nucleus is just one example of the so-called compartmentalization principle underlying the structure of eukaryotic cells. With the help of a complex set of membranes, the cell interior is divided into compartments, like isolated flasks in which various biochemical transformations take place. This "zoning" also greatly increases both the control and effectiveness of a human cell, compared to, for example, a bacterial cell.

Prokaryotic cells are reminiscent of a school for orphans long ago, like that described in *Jane Eyre*: many students of all ages together in one room, working on various subjects, all at the same time. In one corner, they are learning about French verbs, in another they are practicing math, and in a third they are reading a poem, with everyone talking over and distracting one another. It is certainly a way to save money, but it is not a particularly effective system. In nuclear cells, reactions are controlled much like learning processes in a modern school, where the second graders are separate from the fifth graders, everyone learns chemistry in the chemistry lab, and physics experiments are done in the physics room.

In addition to the nucleus, the cytoplasm contains various organelles, that is, "small organs," which allow the cell to carry out various functions, just like "real" organs — the liver, lungs, and brain — perform vital functions for an organism as a whole. Proteins are digested in the lysosomes much like food is digested by the stomach and intestines, while a network of transport microtubules circulates molecules to different parts of the cell, reminiscent of the body's circulatory system. After the nucleus itself, the most important organelle is probably the mitochondria. These are large organelles which act almost as "thermal power plants." They "burn" glucose and provide the cell with the energy it needs in order to support vital processes. At the same time, mitochondria play a major role in regulating programmed cell death, known as apoptosis.

If cells are the building blocks of organisms, then organic molecules are the building blocks of cells. The basic molecules for life – DNA, RNA, proteins – are huge linear polymers, that is, they are "chain" molecules made up of small fragments known as monomers that have been strung together. Because of their size, biological polymers are often referred to as macromolecules. Size matters!

The chemical and physical properties of these large molecules are very different from those of their monomers.

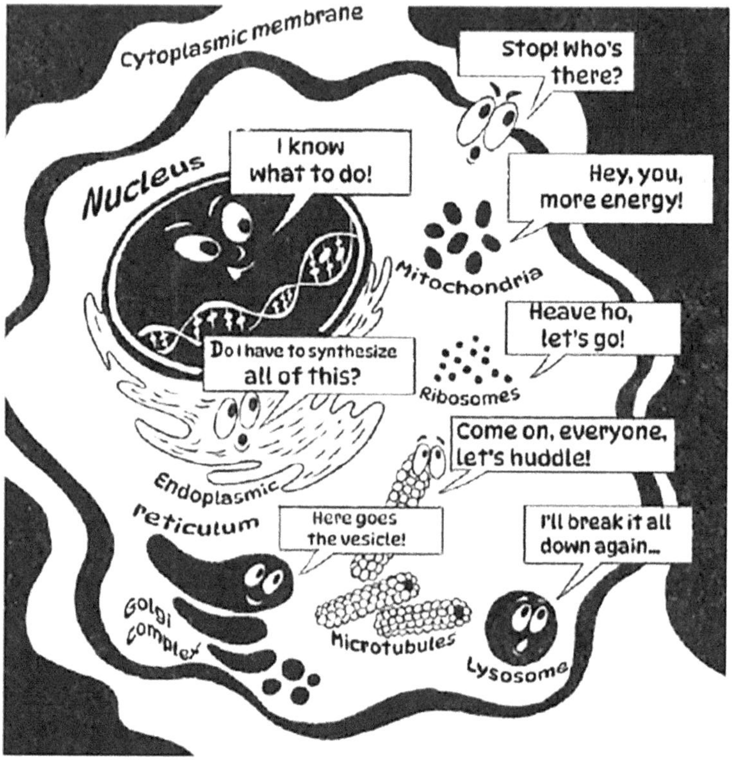

Figure 5. The cell is the basic unit of living material, but its structure is anything but simple! The major cellular organelles were described by cytology researchers in the nineteenth century, though the molecular mechanisms that make them work still hold many mysteries for science.

For example, the polysaccharide cellulose, a hard, insoluble, and poorly digested polymer that forms the basis of wood, is made up of glucose monomers, which are sweet, easily soluble, and edible.

In DNA and RNA, the monomers are organic molecules called nucleotides, while in proteins they are other organic molecules called amino acids (amino acid residues, to be specific). Any linear polymer can be described through the sequence of the monomers of which it is comprised. For example, alanine — glycine — proline — tyrosine — alanine — serine (which can also be recorded as AGPYAS) is the description of a protein fragment. The order in which the amino acid residues are joined together determines the protein's structure and what function it will perform. Genes and RNA molecules, in turn, differ according to the nucleotide sequence.

Biopolymers can be compared to one another, and we can quantify the level of similarity (or difference) between them. For example, the sequences AAAAC and ATAAC differ by only one letter (nucleotide) out of a possible four (A, C, G, and T), so we can say that the degree of homology (similarity) between these two polynucleotides is 80 percent. By comparing the gene sequences of various organisms, scientists collect data on their level of kinship. The more similar the genomes, the more closely related the species are. When studying cancerous tumors, scientists compare the DNA of both cancer cells and healthy cells, which allows them to detect genetic causes of the disease, which we will discuss in more detail below.

Similar analyses allow them to make educated guesses about the structure and functions of poorly understood proteins, by comparing them to well-understood macromolecules. Proteins with sequences that show a high degree of homology (50 percent or higher) generally have similar structures and properties.

Proteins are the main workhorses of the living cell. The human body has just twenty amino acids with various properties — large and small, acidic and alkaline, water-soluble and fatty — but there is a huge number of potential three-dimensional structures that they can build — much like a Lego set, in which a small number of basic blocks can be used to create a wide range of very different constructions.

This multitude of protein structures corresponds to their various functions within the human body. Proteins provide transport and movement, play a role in reproduction and respiration, protect our bodies from infections, and allow us to distinguish between light and darkness. In fact, proteins perform all of the basic tasks in a living cell, with the exception of self-replication. This "smart" molecule cannot synthesize itself. In order to produce proteins, special molecular instructions (written in the DNA) are needed along with special non-protein molecular "synthesizers"—ribosomes (which are based on RNA), which are capable of synthesizing proteins using instructions written in another "nucleotide" language.

FACT: Friedrich Engels was right: Life really is just "the existence of protein bodies"!

THE GENETIC CODE IS BOTH DOGMA AND A ROADMAP!

The three main types of biopolymers — DNA, RNA, and proteins — do not exist outside the body. They are linked together by a relationship that the great scientist Francis Crick described as the "basic dogma of molecular biology." According to this "dogma," genetic information is stored in the cell as a DNA sequence, and carried out in the form of a protein sequence, with the RNA molecule acting as an intermediary for information transfer. The process for recoding a nucleotide sequence into an amino acid takes place on a special molecular machine — a ribosome.

If we were to use a loose computer analogy, DNA can be compared to a program written in a high-level programming language (such as C++). The translation apparatus includes various types of RNA and works as a computer translating the program into a machine code that the computer can understand. We can compare the proteins to an executable file for the resulting game. If one does not know about the principles of compilation, it is almost impossible to detect any sort of link between the source code and the resulting EXE file. This is why it took so long for researchers to notice the relationship between DNA and proteins.

Another, more low-tech analogy might be the link between the recipe for a pie (DNA) and the pie itself (proteins). The cook's skilled hands (ribosomes) transform information hastily jotted down on a scrap of paper into an award-winning pie by combining the necessary ingredients in the right order. But for someone who does not understand what was written down, the relationship between the scrap of paper and the delicacy in front of them may seem like a riddle, if not outright sorcery.

The piece of DNA that encodes the sequence of a particular protein is known as a "gene." All of the genes within a specific organism are known as its genome. This is the first, very rough definition of the molecular basis of life, which will eventually be refined (and become more complicated).

The rules behind the interaction between the DNA sequence and the protein sequence derived from a specific gene are known as the genetic code. The genetic code for all living things on earth is essentially the same, with rare deviations in some bacteria and single-cell organisms, which are exceptions that only confirm the rule. The unity of the genetic code is the main evidence of the common origin of all life forms that we know today.

The genetic code is triplet in nature. This means that one amino acid in a protein is encoded by three nucleotides in the DNA. (We might compare it to the words "one" and "two" in the English language, each of which encodes information in just three letters about the numbers "1" and "2"). The four DNA nucleotides can be used to make up sixty-four triplet codons, which are the main "words" of the genetic alphabet. The majority of these codons encode amino acids. Since there are only twenty amino acids, this means that some amino acids are encoded by several different codons, just as synonyms in one language can all denote the same object or idea. This feature of the genetic code, in which several codons correspond to the same amino acid, is known as degeneracy. Out of the sixty-four codons, three do not code for amino acids. They are known as "stop codons" and their purpose is to stop protein synthesis at the right moment. Stop codons at the end of a sequence encoding proteins act like a period at the end of a sentence.

A substitution in a gene's nucleotide sequence leads to an error (mutation) in the amino acid sequence of a protein, or even the complete cessation of its synthesis in the case of an unplanned appearance of a stop codon at the start of a gene.

Using what you now know, try to solve a problem that sounds fairly simple at first. Each amino acid residue is encoded by three nucleotides; the average length of a protein is about two hundred amino acid residues. How many proteins does the human genome, which measures 3.1 billion base pairs encode (we use "pairs" because the usual DNA structure is a double helix)? Is it really over 5 million?! (3.1 billion ÷ (200 × 3)). The answer is actually only about twenty thousand to twenty-five thousand. But where do we get the enormous discrepancy between the size of the genome and the number of proteins? (Strictly speaking the figures above are not entirely accurate, as a single gene can encode several different proteins, so while the total number of proteins in the human body will be greater than twenty thousand to twenty-five thousand, it will still be far less than 5 million. Each individual cell will only synthesize the parts that correspond to its specialization.)

It turns out that a significant part of the genome is formed by DNA that does not carry any information about proteins. In fact, only about 3 percent of DNA encodes proteins in the human body! And even within genes, the coding pieces of DNA – known as exons – are broken up by non-coding introns. English popular scientist Matt Ridley once rather amusingly compared them to advertising breaking up the text of an interesting article.

Previously, confused researchers dismissed this non-coding part of DNA as "junk DNA," but that view has changed dramatically in the last several years. It turns out that the non-coding DNA plays an important regulatory role, especially in multicellular organisms. Specifically, research has shown that the complexity of an organism (for example, the difference between a human and a worm) has a weak correlation with the total number of genes in the organisms being compared, though there is a convincing correlation with the size of the non-coding genome. That is, the more complex the organism, the more "junk" (or really – regulatory) DNA it will have.

This and other revelations have shed light on our ideas about genes and the genome. Currently, they can be summarized as follows: A cell's genome is formed by the totality of its DNA. The genome's job is to store the information needed for the normal functioning of the proteins necessary for the life of the cell. This information consists of two parts. The first part carries information about a protein's correct sequence of amino acids, which determines its three-dimensional structure and biological function. This information is carried by the coding regions of the corresponding gene. When we match the genome's nucleotide sequence with a specific protein—"protein gene N"—this is what we are referring to. The second part is information on regulating this protein's activities within the cell — when and how much will be read from the gene, whether or not the gene will be active in all cell types or only some of them, and what factors will influence its activity (this is also known as "gene expression"). Somehow (we do not yet fully understand how), this information is stored in the non-coding, regulatory part of the genome.

FACT: Proteins are the building blocks of life, and information about proteins is encoded by genes. Errors in the genome disrupt the normal production of certain proteins, which can change the properties of the cell. For example, a normal cell can turn cancerous.

THE GENOME STRUCTURE IS NO ACCIDENT

Often, descriptions of the human genome in textbooks look like a collection of unrelated facts. However, each component of this complicated system is a part of the solution to a specific and very complex bioengineering task — preserving an organism's genetic material.

Just imagine — the average length of DNA in a human cell is about two meters, while the average cell measures ten to one hundred micrometers (1 micrometer = 0.000001 meter). That means that each cell in our bodies needs to pack the thinnest molecular thread into a tiny volume, without tangling it up or tearing it. Try a similar experiment with a few meters of silk thread, and you will understand how difficult this is.

The DNA molecule contains many active chemical groups — phosphate residues, hydroxyls, amino groups — which are capable of various reactions, and the intracellular environment in which it resides is a very energetic chemical "broth." How can the polymer avoid being damaged in such a difficult environment?

Most importantly, though — the genome is not simply an encyclopedia of cellular information destined to "sit on the shelf" waiting to occasionally be read. Rather, it is a "technical manual" for the cell's day-to-day existence. It is always putting one part or another to work, or running protein synthesis. It is not enough to pack DNA in tight, protect it from undesirable influences, and "put it away in storage." In order for it to continue working properly, it has to effectively interact with the cell and regulate the cell's vital functions, turning various genes "on" and "off." And of course, let us not forget — living cells reproduce by dividing themselves, which means that they are able to preserve the "self-similarity" of all cells in a multicellular organism. In each case, the genome of the mother cell must first be copied and then evenly distributed between two new cells, known as daughter cells. Fulfilling these conditions in the biological systems requires a built-in, complex, and hierarchical genome organization.

If we start with the basics, we have the chemical formula for DNA, which consists of a sequence of nucleotide monomers. We already know that in addition to DNA, living cells contain another nucleic acid known as RNA, which, in the evolutionary sense, is considered by scientists to be DNA's "older sister," having appeared much earlier. RNA has many different (and extremely important) functions within the cell, but storing biological information is not one of them. The genomes of all cellular life forms, from bacteria to human beings, are built only from DNA (with the exception of some viruses). There is much speculation as to why this is the case, but the most plausible explanation is that the different roles of DNA and RNA are related to differences in their molecular structure. The full name for DNA is deoxyribonucleic acid. The ribose sugar in its composition is slightly different compared to that of RNA (ribonucleic acid): rather than a hydroxyl, there is hydrogen in one of the positions, which makes the molecule less flexible, but more stable. That stability is what allowed DNA to win over RNA in the molecular competition and become the main gatekeeper of genetic information in the unimaginably ancient and most likely pre-cellular world.

The primary possibility for saving and copying genetic information is already in the spatial structure of this unusual polymer, which, in the cell, is never represented by a single thread, but is always in the shape of a helix made up of two rows of molecules facing different directions but matching, or, as scientists say, "complementing" one another in order to form a beautiful, symmetrical, and stable structure. Scientists James Watson and Francis Crick received the Nobel Prize for predicting and describing that structure.

Recanceetry of DNA's spatial structure is achieved by the fact that the smaller thymine (T) and cytosine (C) residues always stand opposite the larger adenine (A) and guanine (G) residues, respectively.

Stability is achieved by the fact that residues with similar properties always pair (A–T, G–C), forming either two or three hydrogen bonds, so that no opportunity to form bonds is wasted. Moreover, by stacking the massive and hydrophobic (fatty, literally "fear of water") nucleotides carefully within the helix and exposing the polar, "water-friendly" phosphoric acid residue molecules, DNA is also able to increase its stability. The principle of complementarity means that once we know the sequence of one (any) DNA strand, we can always complete its second, complementary strand. This is exactly what happens during cellular division, when the genetic information is doubled.

Right now, though, it is more important for us to understand how DNA's helical structure helps to preserve genetic information. On one hand, it isolates nucleotides (the sequence of which is actually the significant, "coding" part of the polymer) within the helix, thereby protecting them from chemical influences and modifications. On the other hand, any "irregularity" in the pairing of any "unsuitable residues," such as A–C or C–C, will immediately violate the helix's regular structure and can easily be detected and corrected.

The large number of phosphoric acid residues means that a DNA molecule in water has a negative "acid" charge, and in order to compensate for that and bring the molecule to a more "neutral" and therefore less chemically active state, the cell will use special proteins known as histones, which are rich in positively charged "alkaline" amino acid residues, forming a protein–DNA complex known as a nucleosome. The DNA helix is wound onto the nucleosome ball, forming a structure that has been described by biologists as "beads on a string." These beads are then packed into a denser structure known as a fibril. The fibril is then rolled up and twisted and as a result forms chromatin, a complex made up of DNA and proteins, which allows hereditary information to be packed up densely and in an orderly fashion, while chromatin protein molecules also reliably protect the fragile DNA molecules from interacting with damaging factors. At the same time, various parts of the cellular chromatin might be packed at different densities. Genes that are active in any given type of cell will be found in the areas of loose chromatin, where they are available for interaction with proteins, while the more "dormant genes" will be more densely packed.

When a cell divides, the chromatin of the nucleus is assembled into chromosomes. Each chromosome is a separate strand of DNA, packed as tightly as possible with proteins, and carrying a specific set of genes. Bacterial cells only have one circular chromosome, but most multicellular organisms are based on genomes containing several linear chromosomes. If we were to compare it to books, a bacterial genome is a single volume, while a human genome is a whole "collection of works" with twenty-three volumes, or pairs of chromosomes.

In each cell of the human body (with the exception of sperm and egg cells), this "collection of essays" is present in duplicate – for a total of twenty-three pairs of chromosomes. One chromosome in each pair comes from the maternal egg, and one comes from the paternal sperm. This double or, as scientists say, "diploid" set of genes is also very important. Why? The answer is still the same – to preserve information. If you have two editions of Dumas's *The Three Musketeers* at home, and your dog chews one of them up, you can still read the story to the very end by picking up the second edition. This is the same for cells – duplicating genes increases the "safety margin" and makes it possible to counteract any damage or accidents.

Though genetic information is stored in DNA, the quality of that storage depends on the proteins that control the accuracy of DNA copying (replication) during cell division, and "repair" any genes that happen to contain errors. These proteins form systems or pathways to DNA repair, and there are about ten such pathways in a cell. Repair system proteins literally "scan" a chromosome, and when they detect an error – perhaps an unpaired base, or a break in the chain, or some other alteration that violates the perfect double helix structure – they fix it. Fixing the damage in the sequence leads to restoring the DNA structure. There are several control systems within a cell, and each one is most sensitive to a specific type of error (improper base pairing, a single-strand DNA break, double-strand breaks, etc.), though their functions partially overlap, which makes the repair systems capable of replacing and backing one another up, greatly increasing the cell's genetic stability. Damage to these control proteins leads to genome disorders that are not eliminated in time and begin to accumulate. This is exactly what is observed in certain types of cancer.

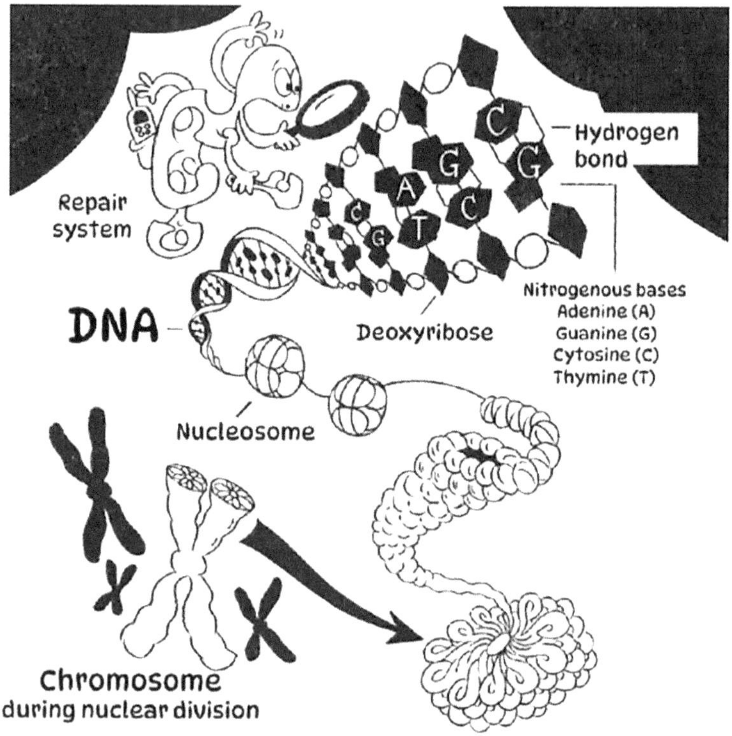

Figure 6. The cell's genome has a complex spatial structure. Histone proteins play an important role in its formation, as they help pack the long molecular strand formed by the DNA double helix into a compact structure, known as the chromosome. Repair system proteins monitor the preservation of DNA and repair any damage. Disruption to this repair process plays an important role in the formation of genomic instability, which is one of the key features of cancer (see Figure 1).

FACT: The human genome is well-protected from damage. But no biological defense is perfect, and there are reasons for that.

The world of RNA

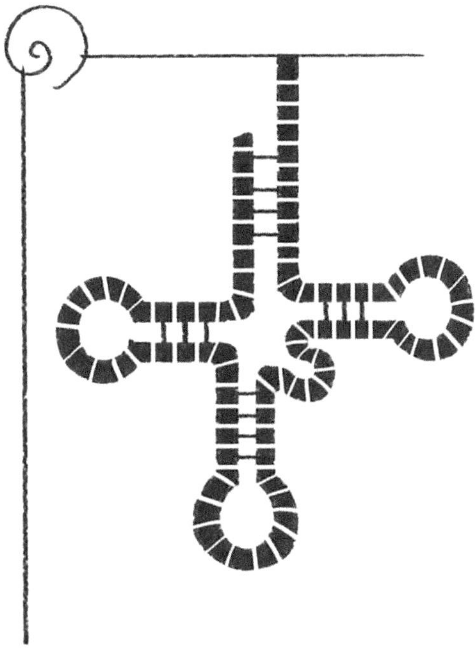

In this book, we will spend a lot of time talking about genes (DNA) and proteins, but very little discussing RNA, as it is impossible to grasp the immensity and include all of the advancements in molecular biology over the past fifty years in one small book. However, at least in this "lyrical digression," we would like to offer a well-deserved tribute to the second nucleic acid, especially because one of the most beautiful molecular biological hypotheses, formulated after the "Central Dogma of Molecular Biology," is the hypothesis of the "world of

RNA," which explains the origin of the three main types of macromolecules — proteins, DNA, and RNA.

The main key to understanding the possible path to life (or rather, "pre-life") at the molecular level has long been that the functions of storing and implementing genetic information in modern organisms are assigned to two very different classes of molecules— DNA and proteins. However, the likelihood that so many different macromolecules were formed randomly in a pre-cellular organic broth is too negligible to be taken seriously. It seems much more plausible that at the origins of pre-life, there was some single group of macromolecules that combined the ability to store and implement information (for example, by synthesizing their own copies). But what kind of substance was this?

Searching for the "progenitor molecule" forced researchers to focus on RNA, which was overshadowed by the other two, better-known macromolecules for a long time. RNA's ability to store genetic information was revealed during a study on viruses. This molecule is less stable than DNA, but at the dawn of the biological era, rapid variability (and therefore the ability to evolve) was probably an advantage, rather than a disadvantage. In 1967, Carl Woese, Francis Crick, and Leslie Orgel were the first to suggest that RNA might be more than simply a repository for genetic information, but also a catalyst molecule capable of speeding up chemical reactions. This assumption was based on the fact that RNA can form a complex spatial structure that is more similar to that of proteins (many of which are catalysts) than DNA's usual structure of a perfect helix "stick." That assumption was later confirmed experimentally, and in 1989 scientists Thomas Cech and Sidney Altman won the Nobel Prize in Chemistry for the discovery of RNA's catalytic properties.

RNA catalysts became known as "ribozymes." While researching hypotheses about the possible origin of life, scientists were able to create artificial RNA polymerase ribozymes capable of catalyzing their own duplication under certain conditions, which perfectly corresponds to the scientists' assumptions about how the progenitor molecule should behave.

Thus, according to modern ideas, the evolution of the pre-cellular molecular broth proceeded as follows: somehow (we still do not know), nucleotides (monomers — the structural units of RNA) were formed from the primary "organic broth," and then joined together to form RNA molecules. Some of these random macromolecules had the ability to reproduce themselves and began to evolve, "competing" with other molecules for limited nucleotide resources. Gradually, they formed entire ensembles of catalytic RNA, which worked together and eventually specialized their functions.

Accumulating random mutations led to the emergence of RNA molecules that catalyze protein synthesis. The proteins turned out to be more effective catalysts than the "parent" RNA, and these mutations became fixed by natural selection. On the other hand, some RNA molecules lost the hydroxyl in their sugar component and turned into DNA, and only stored genetic information. Thus, long before the emergence of the first cells, the modern biochemical world based on DNA and proteins appeared, and RNA lost its leading role, though it continued to act as an intermediary molecule (messenger RNA, or mRNA) and as a regulator of a range of very important and likely ancient processes, such as protein synthesis. Protein-synthesizing ribosome organelles consist of RNA and protein molecules, but it is RNA that performs the catalytic function of joining amino acid residues to the growing protein chain.

Over the last several years, researchers have increasingly focused on the non-coding parts of the genome we described earlier in this book. It turns out that many of them are not quite as non-coding as previously thought. In the human genome, scientists have identified many parts that encode RNA that is not translated into proteins. These untranslated RNA molecules play a major role in regulating many cellular processes, including those associated with cancer.

HEREDITY AND VARIABILITY: WHY WE NEED MUTATIONS

The human genome's protection system is extremely sophisticated and effective, and though it significantly reduces the likelihood of molecular errors, it cannot completely eliminate the possibility of damage.

Errors, or more accurately, "changes" in the genome are called mutations. They can appear at any level of the genome, based on its hierarchical structure.

Some mutations will only affect one or a few nucleotides — the molecular "letters" of the genetic alphabet. These are known as "point mutations," while others, known as gene mutations, will disrupt large fragments of genes. Others damage entire chromosomes and, finally, there are genomic mutations, which change the number of chromosomes in a cell. One such mutation is known as Down Syndrome, in which there are not two copies of chromosome 21 in the genome as there should be, but three.

As we mentioned previously, our genome stores information about the amino acid sequence of each protein as well as the peculiarities of regulating its activities. Mutations in the coding part of a gene can lead to changes in the structure of the protein and affect its ability to perform its functions. A classic example of this type of mutation is damage to the hemoglobin protein in cases of sickle cell anemia, caused by the replacement of one amino acid residue. A mutation in the regulatory part of the genome can result in a protein that has a normal amino acid sequence but is synthesized in greater (or lesser) amounts than necessary, which also disrupts the cell's normal vital functions.

In addition to the amount of genetic material affected by the mutation (one gene or an entire chromosome), it also matters what type of cell — somatic or germinal — is disrupted. Somatic cells are all cells in the human body with the exception of germ cells (sperm and egg cells). A mutation that occurs in the somatic cell will only affect that cell itself and its descendants (if the cell continues to divide despite the damage). Other cells in the body will remain healthy and can compensate for their damaged neighbor's defects. It is quite a different story when the mutation of an important gene or even chromosome takes place in a germ cell — then, the embryo, which is formed by a mutated egg or sperm cell will carry that disorder in all cells of its body (including its germ cells). These mutations are known as congenital mutations, and they are responsible for the appearance of most diseases we describe as "hereditary." One example of this is hemophilia, a disease passed down through the female line (the mutation that causes the disease is present in the X chromosome). People with hemophilia are born with impaired blood clotting, and even a minor wound can cause serious blood loss. One famous person with hemophilia was Tsarevich Alexei in the Russian Empire, who apparently inherited the defective chromosome from his mother Alexandra, whose family had multiple cases of hemophilia.

With age, mutations tend to accumulate in the germ cells, which leads to a heightened risk of genetic abnormalities in children born to older parents. Previously, the medical community tended to wring its hands exclusively over the age of the mother, but in recent years, research has shown that the father's age also plays a significant role in the formation of a healthy embryo. Society currently gives a green light to men who put off having children "for later," despite this being in serious contradiction with his biological nature, and sooner or later may turn out to be the source of both medical and social problems.

Mutations in the somatic cells in sexual reproduction are not inherited, though if people could reproduce by splitting in two, that would be another matter altogether! However, as we will see later on, somatic mutations are only "harmless" to a certain extent — after all, they are the main cause of malignant transformation.

As this book is mainly focused on genome abnormalities that lead to the appearance of cancer, readers may get the wrong idea that all mutations are a bad thing. That could not be further from the truth. Mutations mean change. And changes can be both bad and very good. Evolution creates new species and improves existing ones through a very inefficient but also very effective method — trial and error. For life to evolve, living systems need to inherit heredity — the ability to preserve genetic material and pass it on to their offspring — as well as variability — a less-than-one-hundred-percent accuracy in that preservation and transmission. The measure of variability is the mutation rate, and it may give offspring new features that did not exist before in that species, such as darker skin in order to better withstand hot climates, or the ability to digest milk not only in infancy but also in adulthood, which is a feature absent in animals but present in most humans. The mutation process is like playing roulette, but sometimes, we can win.

The material for a species' natural selection and evolution is primarily the variability of sperm and egg cells. However, given that genome protection mechanisms are the same in all human cells, the price we pay for this ability to evolve is the risk of somatic mutations, some of which lead to the development of cancer.

Scientists now believe that all of modern humanity is descended from a small group of people who left Africa. The human diversity we see today — light and dark skin, statuesque and petite, curly and straight hair — is the result of the uneven accumulation of mutations in different human groups, that is, the fruit of evolution. And even unpleasant things, such as cancer and hereditary diseases, are the essence of the "evolutionary" price vertebrates pay for their great achievements — a well-developed brain and greater life expectancy, which also once looked like "errors" compared to the earlier genetic programming of our worm-like ancestors.

FACT: Genome abnormalities present not only a danger, but also great potential for development. They are our "evolutionary payment" for the ability to evolve and become more sophisticated. Unfortunately, because breaking something down is not the same as building it up, the chance of a single person getting a harmful mutation is much higher than the likelihood of getting a useful change.

CELLULAR DIVISION INEVITABLY LEADS TO GENETIC ERRORS

In 2015, one of the world's most respected scientific journals, *Science*, published an article describing cancer as a disease of "bad luck." Having analyzed all possible tissue systems in the body from the perspective of the likelihood of a malignant tumor developing in them, American researchers demonstrated that the probability of developing a tumor clearly correlates with the number of cellular divisions that have taken place in the tissue since it was formed. Tissues that frequently divide (for example, the epithelium of the stomach or mammary gland ducts) have a higher risk of developing a tumor. Regardless of any other factors, the natural process of cellular division itself is a cancer risk factor.

In the next chapter, we will look more closely at the molecular mechanisms of cellular division but, for now, let us limit ourselves to stating a fact — the more frequently a cell divides, the greater the probability that one of its descendants will have a mutation in the genome. Copying the "genetic text" is just like copying a literary text — mistakes simply happen. Biological systems are incredibly accurate when it comes to copying. For example, erroneous base mutation occurs with a frequency of just 10^{-8} to 10^{-10}, but we must keep in mind that the text is very large, and no matter how hard repair system proteins try to "proofread" all of the DNA — just as in ancient times diligent scribes checked each letter of the Bible or Koran — one way or another, mistakes will still find their way into the "sacred text" of our genome, and in some cases, this will lead to cancer.

The processes for growth and reproduction are distinctive and the most obvious features of living things. They are the first things that come to mind when we compare the "living" and "non-living." Cellular division can be considered as the smallest unit, a sort of "quantum of life." It turns out that this process, even without any outside factors, is a "natural mutagen" capable of causing malignant cellular transformation. Thus, cancer transformation is not so much an aberration as it is an inevitable consequence of the most natural and normal order of things! It is a disconcerting observation, as the logical conclusion is that no human can believe that they are completely safe from the risk of developing a malignant tumor.

There is, however, a silver lining to all of this disturbing news — often, cancer patients find themselves trapped by misconceptions about the cause-and-effect relationship, and torture themselves with unproductive questions such as, "How is this my fault? What did I do wrong?" Unfortunately, this mindset is often sustained by those around them—"A tumor doesn't just appear out of nowhere; it's your own fault!" They will say this as they attempt to assuage their own fears of disease and death with this fallacy. In psychology, this type of bias is known as the "just-world hypothesis." People who share this view believe that the world is set up fairly, and in life we all get what we deserve — good people will be rewarded, and bad people will be punished. At first glance, this worldview may appear to be optimistic, but the other side of this thirst for justice "at any cost" is that the victim (whether of disease or violence) is accused of being guilty for their own suffering.

But that is simply not the case. Even when a person has blatantly ignored their own health for years or has been the victim of someone else's mistakes (for example, radiation exposure after an accident), there is no speaking of blame when it comes to cancer. Cancer is simply a case of misfortune, and it can happen to anyone.

FACT: The main and unavoidable source of mutations is the natural process of cell division.

THE WIDE RANGE OF MUTAGENS

In addition to intracellular mechanisms that determine the "natural" and unavoidable level of errors in our genome, there are also many external factors that can significantly increase the number of mutations. These external factors are known as mutagens. The vast majority of mutagens are also known today as carcinogens — that is, they can cause cancer.

There are many ways to damage the human genome. The DNA–protein complex is a material, physical object, and like any material, physical object, it can be destroyed. Moreover, DNA is an active molecule that is capable of chemical reactions and changing its properties in response to other substances. Finally, the genome of one biological object can be damaged by direct or indirect interaction with another biological object. Thus, we can identify at least three groups of mutagens — physical, chemical, and biological.

Of the physical mutagens, ionizing radiation is the most dangerous. Many physicists who studied radiation during the first half of the twentieth century died of cancer, before radiation's potential danger became clear. Fortunately, the risk of exposure to ionizing radiation is extremely low in most people's everyday lives. But there is another physical factor that can disrupt the structure of DNA, and it is something that we all encounter every day — ultraviolet radiation from the sun. In small doses, ultraviolet rays can even be good for the human body and stimulate vitamin D production. However, in their quest for the perfect tan, many people have literally fried themselves in the sun, and as a result, they accumulated mutations in their skin cells. Ultraviolet light causes the formation of "cross-links" in the DNA molecules, which prevent them from functioning normally. The most common photodamage to DNA is the formation of a dimer between two adjacent thymine residues on the same DNA strand. Doctors attribute rising skin cancer rates (especially melanoma) over the last few decades to the fashion for tanning. By using sunscreen, we can help avoid this danger.

Every now and then, social media begins buzzing over a cancer "epidemic" caused by other physical factors (such as microwave ovens or cell phone radiation), but to date, there is no conclusive evidence that electromagnetic radiation from household appliances has any significant effect on cancer risk.

Chemical mutagens include substances with a variety of different structures. Special precautions must be taken when using mutagenic (carcinogenic) substances, and in most countries, their widespread use in homes is usually prohibited or severely restricted by law. Carcinogenic substances include the products of the combustion of many organic substances, especially petroleum and hard coal. This is why thermal power plants that use this type of fuel must have emission purification systems. Of course, one of the most widespread household carcinogens is cigarette smoke — countless studies have confirmed the link between smoking and a heightened risk of lung, mouth, and throat cancer. Rapid growth in the chemical and pharmacological industry during the second half of the twentieth century led to the question of developing a fast and reliable method for the primary testing of mutagenic potential in new (and existing) chemical compounds. In the end, the Ames test was developed, and has remained in use for many years. The idea behind this test is that mutated bacteria which are unable to synthesize a vital amino acid known as histidine will try to grow in a histidine-poor nutrient medium. The substance being studied will be added to the same medium. If it is non-mutagenic, bacterial colonies will grow very slowly in the poor medium. But if the substance in question happens to be a mutagen, the bacterial colony will likely produce a (reverse) mutation, and once the microorganisms have regained their ability to cope without histidine, they will enthusiastically get back to their favorite activity — reproducing. Of course, a simple test like this is no substitute for more detailed research, and it is possible that a substance that does not act on the bacteria might suddenly show mutagenic effects, for example, on mice, but as a preliminary screening method for potentially dangerous substances, the Ames test continues to be the easiest, cheapest, and most effective.

Speaking of genome abnormalities caused by external factors, we cannot ignore "biological mutagens"—namely, viruses. Many of them are capable of inserting themselves into the human genome and disrupting its normal structure. Others provoke the development of chronic inflammation in the infected tissue, which also heightens the risk of malignancy. For some time now, viruses have been convincingly proven to play a role in the formation of several tumors. Nonetheless, even a cancer caused by a virus is not a "viral" or "infectious" disease in the classical sense. Fortunately, the scientific community is not currently aware of any viruses that "guarantee" the formation of cancer in the same way that, for example, the HIV virus guarantees the development of AIDS. It is known that women infected with some varieties of the human papillomavirus will have higher rates of cervical cancer (more on that later), but there are also many women who have this virus in their body who never get cancer. The same can be said for other cancers of viral origin.

Cancer is not a disease that one can "catch," though you can catch an infection that heightens your risk of cancer developing. We should also keep in mind that even in the unluckiest cases, several years will go by between the time of infection and the development of the cancerous tumor, and by the time the cancer symptoms have appeared, there are likely no longer any traces of the viral infection that caused it. In any case, the risk of contracting cancer-causing viruses is fairly easy to avoid. It is enough to follow some basic hygiene requirements. After all, most viruses that have to date been proven to cause cancer are either sexually transmitted or blood borne. Your chances of contracting them through normal, everyday contacts is almost zero. Unfortunately, a poor understanding of how cancer works has led to terrible situations in many countries where healthy people refuse to let cancer patients be near them, and even collect signatures to evict a mother with a sick child from their apartment buildings because they believe that cancer is a contagious disease. Remember, "the sleep of reason produces monsters." This is completely unacceptable discrimination.

In the early 1900s, American scientist Francis Rous was the first to prove the existence of viruses that were capable of causing cancerous tumors in birds. For a long time, his research was not appreciated on its merits, as it went against the dogma that cancer can only be caused by chemical and physical factors in one's environment. Rous did not receive the Nobel Prize for his scientific discovery until fifty years later in 1966. Nine years after that, in 1975, the Nobel Prize again went to a team of American researchers — David Baltimore, Renato Dulbecco, and Howard Temin — who explained the molecular mechanisms that viruses use to embed themselves into the human genome.

The first description of a virus capable of causing cancerous tumors in humans was in 1965. It was Epstein-Barr virus, which can cause a very rare but very malignant Burkitt's lymphoma (lymphoma is the malignant transformation of one's own immune cells, or lymphocytes; we will discuss them more in Chapter 7). Unlike other lymphomas, this disease is localized in certain geographical regions. It is most common in Central Africa, and rarer in the United States. In Russia, Burkitt's lymphoma is very rare; though infectious mononucleosis, which produces symptoms similar to that of a lingering cold, and which is caused by the virus, is extremely widespread. This demonstrates that the virus is a necessary but certainly not the sole condition for the malignant rearrangement of our immune system cells. Soviet biologist Lev Zilber is considered the Russian founder of the viral theory of cancer. Zilber began his oncology research while serving a prison sentence for anti-Soviet activities and luckily avoided execution. Instead, he was sent to a secret carceral research-and-development institute, where he carried out his first experiments on rats that the prisoners caught for him. After Zilber was released in 1944, his article on the viral nature of cancer was published in *Izvestia*, which was one of the USSR's two main official newspapers. His suspicion about the virus's important role in initiating the malignant transformation process turned out to be very prescient.

Today, it is believed that about 15 percent of cancerous tumors around the world are somehow related to viruses. This category is led by liver cancer in men and cervical cancer in women. German scientist Harald zur Hausen won the Nobel Prize in 2008 for explaining the role of human papillomavirus in the development of cervical cancer. The study of oncoviruses may be one of the most "fruitful" areas of biology when it comes to the number of Nobel Prizes for research.

It is difficult to treat tumors caused by oncoviruses, but many of them can be averted in the first place by preventing infections and through vaccination programs, just as we stave off other viral diseases (measles, whooping cough, smallpox). The first anti-cancer vaccines (against human papillomavirus), Gardasil and Cervarix, are used around the world. These vaccines protect from the most dangerous types of human papillomavirus (types 16 and 18), thereby preventing the occurrence of related cancers, such as cervical, vaginal, and vulval cancer in women, and anal and penile cancer in men. Vaccination is recommended for young people aged nine to twenty-six, ideally before becoming sexually active, as oncogenic papillomaviruses are almost exclusively sexually transmitted. In 2018, the Food and Drug Administration in the United States approved these vaccines for older groups of people. In a group of females aged twenty-seven to forty-five, vaccination provided 88 percent protection from genital warts, precancerous epithelial dysplasia and cervical, vulval, and vaginal cancer.[3] In many countries, these vaccines are included in the national vaccination schedule. In the United States, they are part of the Centers for Disease Control and Prevention's recommended routine vaccination for both

3 https://www.fda.gov/news-events/press-announcements/fda-approves-expanded-use-gardasil-9-include-individuals-27-through-45-years-old.

boys and girls as of ages eleven or twelve, and in the United Kingdom, they are offered to both boys and girls aged twelve to thirteen. In Russia, they are not part of the compulsory vaccination schedule, but can be administered for a fee at medical institutions.

Russian (and other countries') compulsory vaccination schedules do include vaccination against hepatitis B, however. When parents vaccinate their child against this disease, they are protecting them from a serious viral infection as well as liver cancer.

Neither prophylactic measures nor vaccination offer 100 percent guaranteed protection, but together they can significantly minimize the risk of disease.

FACT: Most mutagens are completely unpredictable. To a certain extent, we know how much a specific agent will influence the increased rate of mutation, but we cannot predict which part of the genome will be disrupted in any given case. This is a random process based on probability.

DOES EVERY MUTATION CAUSE CANCER?

People were aware of the presence of hereditary congenital anomalies and effects long before the advent of genetics, let alone molecular biology. Though the majority of these defects are clearly genetic, they have nothing to do with cancer. From the early days of molecular oncology, it was clear that though cancer always involves mutations (and often there are more than one), not every mutation leads to cancer — far from it. It is clear that mutations in some parts of the genome are more carcinogenic than others.

When developments in molecular biology methods made it possible to talk about disorders in a specific gene rather than simply "mutations" in general, biologists rushed to study exactly which genes go through changes in various types of cancer. That work is still ongoing, but it is already obvious that in the vast majority of tumors, dysfunctions in a relatively small number of genes trigger the development of cancer. Other disruptions and genome rearrangements are usually a consequence of these primary mutations.

From a functional standpoint, the genes responsible for tumor development can clearly be divided into two groups — oncogenes (pro-cancer genes) and oncosuppressors (anti-cancer genes)—though in popular medical literature, they are often combined into one general category of "oncogenes," or genes with some sort of relationship to cancer. This generalization is not very accurate.

In order to understand the difference between oncogenes and oncosuppressors in terms of cancer development, we must first speak a bit about the regulation of gene activity in human cells. As you will remember, all cells in our multicellular organism contain the same genome (plus or minus a few somatic mutations accumulated over the course of our lives). Nonetheless, these cells both look and act very differently. A neuron does not resemble a liver cell, and a lymphocyte does not look like a muscle cell. This difference is because different sets of genes are active in different cells, which synthesize different sets of proteins. Controlling the life of the cell, and more broadly the life of the entire multicellular organism, can be described by changing gene activities (expression), which leads to an increase or decrease in synthesis of the proteins they encode.

Oncogenes are genes that are more active in a tumor than in normal, healthy tissue. This result can be achieved by point mutations that change protein activity, or by gene mutations when the number of oncogene copies increases in a cancer cell (amplification), along with the synthesis of the corresponding protein. One example of such an oncogene is the *HER2* (also known as *ERBB2*) gene, which is amplified in some types of breast cancer.

Oncosuppressors are genes and proteins that in normal conditions "insure" a cell against cancerous transformations. Contrary to oncogenes, the function of oncosuppressors in a tumor cell is lower than normal. The most well-known oncosuppressor is the *TP53* gene (and protein), which we will hear about more throughout this book. Usually, the "breakdown" of oncosuppressor genes is what leads to cancer. Mutations in the *TP53* gene can be found in tumors in various organs and appear to be the culprit behind over half of all cancers, though this is not the only oncosuppressor that can break down in a cell.

Regulating processes in a cell can be compared to regulating street traffic. Oncogenes are like daredevil drivers, while oncosuppressors are like strict traffic controllers. The more reckless drivers and the fewer people you have to ensure order on the road, the more likely it is that there will be an accident — or a rebirth of cancerous cells.

Though the concept of oncogenes and oncosuppressors is generally widely accepted, there are still many unanswered questions about the specifics. The p53 protein, which is one of the few "universal" oncosuppressors, is more of an exception than a rule. In most cases, we can see that mutations in various oncogenes and oncosuppressors accompany the development of cancer in various organs. Why does a mutation in the *APC* gene predominate in colon and stomach tumors, while a disruption on the *RB1* gene causes a rare eye tumor known as a retinoblastoma, and a fusion of the *EWS* and *FLI1* genes causes an aggressive Ewing's sarcoma in the tubular bones? Scientists have yet to find any definitive answers to these questions.

A mutation in one or more oncogenes or oncosuppressors generally triggers a malignant tissue transformation, which is known as a "precancerous state," though after this, it will take at least several more cell generations before the healthy tissue finally transforms into cancerous tissue. As a cancerous tumor evolves, it accumulates these new mutations, some of which will gradually aggravate malignant properties in the cells, while others will accompany them as a consequence of the general instability in the genome. The first type of mutation is known as a "driver mutation"—these drive the transformation of healthy tissue into cancerous tissue. The second type is known as a "passenger mutation"—these are not important to the tumor cell's vital activities, but their numbers make it possible for scientists to estimate how far the tumor development has progressed.

Some mutations in oncogenes and oncosuppressors can be inherited, which will determine a family's predisposition to certain types of cancers. The most well-studied disease in this category is a form of breast cancer that depends on mutations in the *BRCA1* and *BRCA2* oncosuppressor genes (we will speak more about this later).

Though the idea of carrying a "cancer gene" is a frightening prospect, we should keep in mind that these forms of cancer only make up a small percentage (about 5 to 10 percent) of all cancer cases. The overwhelming majority of cancer cases are not inherited, but are simply due to mutations acquired over the course of one's life. But if previous generations of your family have had several cases of similar cancers that strike at a young age (before the age of seventy or eighty), perhaps you should consult with a medical genetics specialist to test for a genetic predisposition to the disease. These tests are now readily available based on consultation with your physician. Breast, ovarian, colon, and stomach cancers are the diseases most likely to be influenced by genetic factors.

Sometimes the development and outcome of cancer is compared to Russian roulette, given its unpredictability. This is apt, given its rather grim precision. Whether mutations appear in a given part of the human genome is an unpredictable, random process. There are plenty of cases of chain smokers who manage to live well into old age, while people who have done everything to maintain a healthy lifestyle end up in the oncology ward. However, it is useless to sit around in despair, and it is worth knowing that there are several ways to play Russian roulette. Cancer survival rates greatly depend on how many bullets are in the magazine. One? Two? Maybe even five?

The good news is that the number of "bullets" in the cancer revolver is largely up to us. By limiting our contact with carcinogens and leading a reasonably healthy lifestyle, we can minimize the likelihood of developing cancer. Unfortunately, though, no one is completely immune to what amounts to bad luck at the molecular level.

FACT: Only a small percentage of cellular mutations will lead to cancer. It does not matter what factors (physical, chemical, or biological) triggered the disruption in the genome; when it comes to cancer, the only thing that matters is whether the genes that determine whether a tumor develops — oncogenes and oncosuppressors — are affected.

BRCA — THE "ANGELINA JOLIE GENES"

In 2013, famous Hollywood actress Angelina Jolie had surgery to remove both of her breasts in order to avoid breast cancer. Later on, she had her ovaries removed as well. In the United States, this kind of surgery has long been commonplace, and in this case, the only surprise may have been Jolie's willingness to speak publicly about a topic that most people find difficult and scary.

Jolie's openness was likely a great source of psychological support for the thousands of women around the world who have to undergo this kind of surgery each year. Breast cancer is the most common type of cancer. Generally speaking, though, surgery for this type of diagnosis is to treat rather than prevent cancer. So why would a perfectly healthy young woman decide to go under the knife?

To understand why, we need to go back in time to the 1940s, when, prior to the advent of modern diagnostic methods, English doctor and researcher David Smithers used a good, old-fashioned family tree and published research on the family histories of 450 female patients with breast cancer, demonstrating that in several cases the disease was clearly hereditary, and occurred much more frequently in a family's female line than one would expect based on average cancer rates in the country. In these cases, the cancer developed in women who were younger (before the age of fifty), was more aggressive, and was more difficult to treat.

Smithers' observation was later confirmed by other research, but it was not until the 1980s that scientists were able to identify the gene, or rather pair of genes — *BRCA1* and *BRCA2*-in which mutations were responsible for the development of this type of disease. The abbreviations for the BRCA genes literally stand for "breast cancer."

The genetics of BRCA-dependent cancers turned out to be even more interesting than was previously thought. In order for healthy cells to become tumor cells, a mutation must occur in both copies of the gene. However, if these two mutations take place in the germ cells, they will cause the death of the embryo in the early stages of embryogenesis, due to the high number of genetic abnormalities. The pattern of inheriting a genetic predisposition to this type of cancer is as follows: The carrier of the mutated BRCA gene inherits it, as a rule, from her mother (Angelina Jolie's mother died young of breast cancer), meaning that for her, it is a germline mutation that is present in all cells in her body. The woman inherits a second, healthy gene from her father (remember that in the human genome, genes and chromosomes are present in pairs). The healthy gene compensates for the damaged one, and the woman can live for many years without any type of health issues. However, as she ages, somatic mutations accumulate in her body cells. If, by some unfortunate accident, one of them happens to affect the healthy copy of the BRCA gene, that cell can no longer protect itself from the breakdown in the genome, and it will either die or turn into a cancer cell. There are many cells in the body, and the probability of malignant transformation is high.

The fact that this genetic breakdown is an inherited trait may be the reason behind the fact that cancer rates differ among ethnicities. Asian Americans have lower cancer rates than Americans whose ancestors came from Europe, although differences in lifestyle among various ethnic groups (diet, physical activity) probably play an important role as well. I was unable to find similar statistics for Russia but, based on global experience, I can confidently say that people whose ancestors belong to a small ethnic group that avoided contact with outsiders for centuries should probably take a closer look at their health than those whose ancestors hailed from various regions and ethnic groups.

Research has shown that in closed groups, in which members for various reasons often intermarried, harmful mutations tend to accumulate, which heightens the risk of developing many hereditary diseases, including cancerous tumors. One classic (and very well-studied) example of such a group is Ashkenazi Jews (a subethnic group of Jews who descend from Jewish populations in Central and Eastern Europe who spoke Yiddish). Ashkenazi Jews' common origin from a relatively small, closed population group has had a profound effect on their gene pool and, today, members of this group have a notably increased risk of several genetic diseases, including cancers related to BRCA gene mutations.

Modern molecular diagnostics for patients and their relatives have refined Smithers' statistics. Research revealed that damaged *BRCA1* and *BRCA2* genes contribute to the development not only of breast cancer, but also of ovarian cancer. In women who carry these genes, the risk of falling ill can reach up to 80 percent. This is why in some countries (especially in the United States), doctors recommend removing ovaries and the breast tissue in women with a BRCA defect and a history of cancer in their maternal line, once they have had their desired number of children. In other countries, the approach is less radical and limited to more frequent and deeper screenings of those who carry the gene, in order to catch cancer at its earliest stages. In any case, a woman who is found to carry this genetic defect faces a difficult choice. There is hope that with the advent of a new class of drugs known as PARP inhibitors, the medical field will be able to curb this type of cancer, at least in part. Although BRCA gene mutations present much more of a danger to women's health, they are not without consequence for men. Male carriers of defective genes have a heightened risk of prostate cancer or male breast cancer (yes, males can also get breast cancer), so men whose families have high rates of hereditary breast cancer in the female line would do well to also be tested for BRCA mutations.

FACT: The presence of BRCA gene mutations greatly increases a woman's likelihood of having breast or ovarian cancer. If this cancer is in the female line of your family tree, you should consider genetic testing. If the results show you carry the mutation, you should monitor your health more closely. A BRCA mutation is not a sentence, but it is an aggravating factor.

IF YOU CANNOT BEAT THEM, TAKE CHARGE OF THEM!

One thing that sets apart cancers related to BRCA gene mutations is their marked genetic instability. Every cancerous tumor has mutations (as we already discussed), often numbering in the dozens (this is a lot; a healthy cell only accumulates a few mutations over its life). But the genomes of tumors in which the *BRCA1* gene stops working look frantic. These tumors contain literally every type of genetic disorder: point mutations and changes to the number of gene copies and chromosomes. This is what makes these types of tumors so aggressive and dangerous. By mutating quickly, cells with the disrupted BRCA gene function easily take on new properties, such as a resistance to drugs and accelerated metastasis. This is why this type of cancer does not respond well to traditional treatments (surgery plus chemotherapy). What is causing this type of cellular behavior?

The answer lies in the fact that *BRCA1* and *BRCA2* proteins encoded by the corresponding genes are important components of DNA repair (one almost wants to write "restoration") systems in cells. Damage to the BRCA genes and the proteins they encode leads to a decrease in the quality of DNA being copied in the cell, and more and more new mutations begin to accumulate in it (even without any external mutagens). The same link between damage to the genes encoding proteins responsible for DNA repair and genomic instability was later noted in other types of cancerous tumors.

In a biological system, however, instability is only an advantage up to a certain point. Control mechanisms that ensure genome sustainability in a tumor are often disrupted, but not entirely destroyed, or else the cancer cells would simply die. Malignant cells are able to survive with a greater number of genetic disruptions than normal cells (we will discuss the reasons why later on), but their ability to adapt to these abnormalities is not infinite, either.

As a result of thinking about the relationship between genetic instability and cancer cell survival, researchers came up with the idea of amplifying a tumor's genetic instability to the point that it is incompatible with cell survival. As mentioned above, in normal cells, there are several molecular pathways responsible for DNA repair, and they partially duplicate and support each other's functions. One of them is a function of the proteins encoded by BRCA genes, and is already disrupted in this type of cancer – but what happens if another repair mechanism is turned off in the tumor cells as well? For example, scientists wanted to know what happens if the repair mechanism associated with the PARP protein, responsible for repairing single-stranded DNA, also breaks?

It turns out that if a cancer cell in which BRCA is already disrupted is also exposed to a substance that blocks PARP, the level of genome errors becomes so high that the cell dies. This phenomenon is known as "synthetic lethality." Separately, neither a disruption in the BRCA mechanism nor inhibiting PARP will cause any significant harm to the cancer cell, but the two actions together—"synthetically"—will destroy it. These treatments will also cause less damage to healthy cells than traditional chemotherapy. Interestingly, the effect of PARP inhibitors can also be enhanced, which will warm the tumor somewhat. Temperatures of 41 °C to 42 °C will degrade (destroy) the *BRCA2* protein, the cancer cells will experience worsened DNA repair, and the treatment will have a stronger effect.

A new class of drugs based on PARP inhibitors was recently approved as therapy for cancers associated with BRCA mutations and have proven themselves to be highly effective in treating patients.

FACT: PARP inhibitors are one example of a highly specialized, "targeted" drug that is effective for a specific group of tumors related to disruptions in the BRCA genes.

SUMMARY

In this chapter, we learned that cancer is a disease of the genome that is always caused by mutations in certain genes — oncogenes and oncosuppressors — and that these mutations lead to general genomic instability, manifested by the fact that in many (if not all!) cancer cells, there are high numbers of point mutations and chromosomal rearrangements. The causes of this genetic transformation are diverse — physical, chemical, or biological.

It is possible to inherit mutations in oncogenes and oncosuppressors, which creates a hereditary predisposition to some types of disease, though "hereditary" cancers are only 5 to 10 percent of all cases. The main cause of cancer is an individual's own somatic mutations, which are accumulated during the course of one's life, rather than "bad" genes inherited from one's ancestors. However, if your family history suggests a hereditary tendency to cancer, it is a good idea to look into genetic testing.

One classic example of an inherited cancer is breast and ovarian cancer in women who carry BRCA gene mutations. The proteins encoded by these genes are usually responsible for one of the DNA repair pathways in case of an accidental breakage. When the BRCA protein function is disrupted, this leads to the genome starting to accumulate new damage and becoming unstable. In recent years, the medical community has seen a breakthrough in treating this type of cancerous tumor. There is a new approach, which involves using PARP inhibitors, suggesting that if several DNA repair pathways are blocked simultaneously within a cancer cell, this will bring the number of genetic errors to a high level no longer compatible with the tumor's survival.

Along with this new knowledge, we also have new questions. Cancer is always the result of disruption in the genome, but why is not every genome disorder cancer? We have figured things out with the *BRCA1* protein. But how do the proteins of other oncogenes and oncosuppressors work?

Later on in this book, we will discuss the relationship between genome disorders and disruptions in normal cellular life processes as well as the prospects for new cancer treatment therapies.

Chapter 3
CELL DIVISION SECRETS AND MYTHS ABOUT CHEMOTHERAPY

Despite the advent of so many new and targeted cancer drugs, the most common methods of cancer treatment are still surgery, radiation (radiotherapy), and traditional chemotherapy. Unfortunately, when it comes to cancer, a spoonful of sugar will most certainly not make the medicine go down. Due to its numerous side effects, many people believe that "chemo" is worse than cancer itself — that the treatment is worse than the disease. This idea is not entirely wrong, either. Indeed, there are cases in which chemo is inadvisable, due to the patient's advanced age or the presence of other serious and concomitant diseases, so physicians will look for other ways to treat these patients' cancer.

However, in most cases, chemotherapy drugs can significantly improve the effect of surgery and stave off the development of inoperable forms of cancer. In order to understand how chemotherapy works and why it causes the side effects that it does, we need to understand how the cell cycle works. We will also discuss a new generation of drugs that block cancer cell division at the level of the signaling pathways while also causing fewer unpleasant side effects than traditional chemotherapy.

CHEMOTHERAPY – FOLLY OR NECESSITY?

Chemotherapy, often referred to simply as "chemo," is one of oncology's "boogeymen." When people go through chemo, they suffer from nausea, they lose their appetite, their hair falls out, and they have stomach and intestinal bleeding. It might seem like a treatment that consists of nothing but nasty side effects, with no guarantee of a recovery, and it is no coincidence that cancer patients and their relatives often ask, "Why bother?" after seeing their loved ones in anguish. People rarely doubt the necessity of surgery for cancer treatment. But when it comes to chemo… is it really necessary? Unfortunately, it is.

For a long time, the only treatment for cancerous tumors was surgery. If something "extra" was growing on you, you would cut it off. But from the early days of surgical cancer treatments, doctors noticed that different types of tumors did not have the same reaction to surgery. Sometimes they were destroyed entirely and never returned, while others would come back time and again, spread throughout the body, and eventually kill the patient. Thus, tumors were empirically divided into "benign" and "malignant." Later on, with the advent of cytological methods, it became clear that benign tumor cells look different under a microscope than malignant ones, and therefore tumors could be classified without waiting to see whether or not they returned.

During the twentieth century, cancer surgery made progress in leaps and bounds. For example, it became clear that surrounding tissue had to be removed along with the tumor, as it might contain cancer cells that are invisible to the naked eye. New instruments and tools were also developed, making it possible to operate on organs that doctors were previously unable to access, though the modernization of surgical interventions itself did not significantly improve cancer patients' life expectancy.

There was, however, some progress in this area once doctors began treating patients with a combination of surgery and radiation therapy, or radiotherapy.

Radiation causes more damage to cells that are dividing than cells that are at rest, and radiation therapy involves irradiating the tumor via ionizing radiation (alpha particles, neutrons, protons, etc.), and is still a common treatment for malignant tumors. In some cases, radiation therapy (in which a beam of ionizing radiation is aimed at a specific location in the body) is the only possible treatment (for example, in cases involving brain tumors). However, this method is far from a panacea, and leads to many negative side effects comparable to those of chemotherapy, the most serious of which is the carcinogenic effect of ionizing radiation, which we discussed in the previous chapter.

Most of oncology's success during the twentieth and early twenty-first centuries has been related to the advent of more-targeted diagnostic methods and the development of pharmacological treatments for malignant tumors. The introduction of the drug cisplatin is just one example of this. With cisplatin, the five-year survival rate for testicular cancer without any recurrence jumped from 10 percent to 85 percent — and this is just one drug and one specific type of cancer.

Sometimes, when patients are diagnosed early on, they do not have to undergo chemo — this is one argument to convince you and your loved ones to be vigilant when it comes to monitoring your health — but at later stages, there is simply no way to avoid surgery and medication. Today, oncologists have dozens, if not hundreds, of medications in their arsenal, and it is hard to imagine a time when treating cancer with drugs was simply unthinkable. After all, malignant tumors were (and still are) notoriously challenging targets for any pharmaceutical treatment.

Sometimes, people believe that tumors are hard to kill. In fact, it is not difficult at all to kill a cancerous tumor *in vitro* (outside the body, in an artificial environment, usually in a lab). If the goal of pharmacological science was simply to "destroy the tumor"—it would have been attained long ago. But in fact, the goal of destroying the tumor while leaving the patient alive is far more difficult, and therein lies the challenge. All of the most effective drugs aimed at fighting invaders in our bodies, whether antibiotics or drugs for parasitic worms, play on genetic and molecular differences between the cells of the parasite and those of the host. For example, popular antibiotics such as streptomycin and gentamicin work because they bind to bacterial cell ribosomes, thereby disrupting protein synthesis. Prokaryotic ribosomes differ from eukaryotic ribosomes, and these antibiotics are almost harmless to human cells.

However, a cancer cell's genetic and molecular "portrait" is nearly identical to that of a normal cell, and for a long time, scientists struggled with how to destroy a tumor without also destroying the organism. The advent of chemotherapy was in fact as accidental as the discovery of antibiotics. I would describe it as a "happy accident," but that seems inappropriate given that this discovery stems from what would later be categorized as a war crime.

FACT: Cancer cells are very similar to normal, healthy cells, which means that it is very difficult to create a medication that will destroy the tumor cells without causing significant harm to the organism.

CHEMO AND LIFE

Classical chemotherapy was begat on the battlefields of World War I. There, near the Belgian town of Ypres, was where the German Army first deployed a chemical warfare agent known as "mustard gas." At the dawn of the twentieth century, Germany was the world's leading chemical power. Unfortunately, some discoveries by German chemists were so-called "dual-use" technologies, including mustard gas, which caused serious damage to the eyes, skin, and respiratory tract, inflicting pain and suffering on the victim for months. By studying soldiers who had been poisoned, doctors discovered decreased levels of white blood cells and a sharp drop in the rate of bone marrow (the body's main hematopoietic — that is, blood-forming — tissue) cell division. This meant that the poison had an effect on the cells that divided the most actively, without any noticeable damage to the rest of the body.

This also explained why it took victims so long to recover from mustard gas attacks — after all, healing from wounds requires cells in the surrounding tissue to divide more rapidly. During the World War I era, doctors usually observed this cytostatic effect as a method for diagnosing mustard gas poisoning. However, during the 1940s, American researchers Louis Goodman and Alfred Gilman hypothesized that at just the right dosage, the poison (or rather, its derivatives) could be used to effectively kill cancer cells. After all, accelerated and chaotic proliferation (division) is the hallmark of a malignant tumor. The "genetic" definition of cancer we examined in the previous chapter becomes much more precise when we add in a reference to this key biological process: "Cancer is a disease of the genome which leads to excessive activation of cellular division."

The first clinical trials of this new drug followed soon after. (At the time, academic and medical ethics were very different from those in place today, and it was quite common for doctors to conduct experiments on their patients. Strict protocols requiring preclinical studies on medical drugs did not come about until much later.) A patient diagnosed with lymphosarcoma and identified only by the initials J. D. went down in medical history when he was injected intravenously with the first dose of poison. On the fourth day of chemotherapy, the tumor decreased, and a week later, his external symptoms entirely disappeared. Within a month, J. D.'s cancer had gone into remission — blood tests revealed no cancer cells were present.

A few years later, another American researcher, Sidney Farber, demonstrated that by using folic acid antagonists he was able to reverse the frantic blood cell division seen in leukemia patients. Folic acid, which is a necessary vitamin for normal hematopoiesis, had been discovered in a study on a form of anemia. In healthy people, folic acid helps support normal blood cell production. But in patients with leukemia — a "blood cancer" that causes immature blood cells to divide abnormally fast and literally "clog" the blood vessels while being incapable of fulfilling their normal functions — taking folic acid sharply exacerbated the disease. Farber suggested that the action of substances that block folic acid activity (antifolates) might help leukemia patients. In 1947, Farber gave the first injection of antifolates to a two-year-old patient who was dying of acute leukemia. The first version of the drug did not have any noticeable effect on the child, but the second version of the antagonist molecule, known as amethopterin, quickly brought the disease into remission. Within a few days, the number of cancerous leukoblast cells in the blood dropped several times, and the child regained his strength and appetite. This was the beginning of modern chemotherapy, though it took several decades of careful lab work to understand why this group of drugs is so selective when it comes to dividing cells. The key to understanding the molecular mechanisms behind chemotherapy was the study of the cell cycle — that is, the time interval from one cellular division to the next.

CELL CYCLE OR LIFE CYCLE?

The life of most human body cells can be divided into several periods — or phases — each of which includes specific events that take place to prepare the cell for reproduction and ensure division.

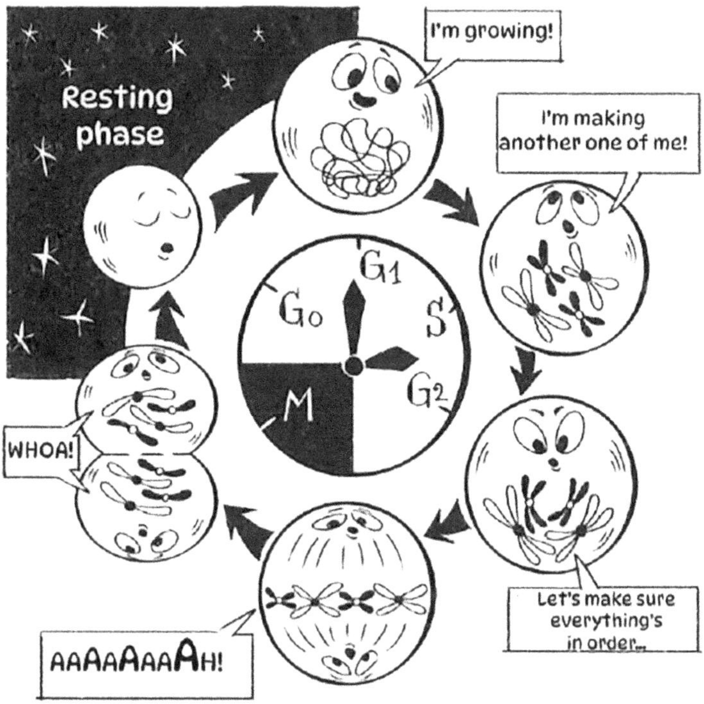

Figure 7. The cell cycle, or the period from one cell division to the next, looks like a wheel. In cancer cells, this wheel moves unusually fast (see Figure 1).

Although cells "work" differently in different tissues of our bodies, they all divide in more or less the same way. The molecular mechanisms of this key life process are very conservative, which is why sometimes the same chemo medications are used to treat different types of tumors.

The first phase of the cell cycle is known as G0 (G stands for gap), or the resting phase, during which the cells do not divide. Some types of cells, for example neurons or heart muscle cells, enter the resting phase once they have reached maturity and remain in that state forever, but for other cells, this period is like a pause between two divisions. The longer a cell is at rest, the less often it will divide, and vice versa — in cancer cells, the G0 phase is usually very short, as they move from one reproduction cycle to the next quite literally "without stopping to breathe."

Chemotherapy drugs are developed based on substances that will cause minimal damage to cells in the G0 phase, but which are active against cells that are no longer at rest. This is how doctors can at least partially reduce the side effects related to the fact that chemotherapy's toxicity will affect any dividing tissues, at least to some degree.

A cell that is about to divide leaves the G0 phase and enters the preparatory G1 phase. Division requires a high number of resources, which need to be prepared in advance. During the G1 phase, the cell will increase in size and produce the RNA and proteins necessary to synthesize DNA during the division process. The G1 phase is an especially important step in the cell cycle, because this is when the cell still has the ability to "change its mind." If, for some reason, the cell does not divide, it will leave the G1 phase and return to a resting state. In later stages, there is usually no more "turning back," and the cell will have to either complete the division process or die off. Once the cell has reached the necessary size, and the proteins it needs have been synthesized, it will enter the next phase in the cycle, known as the S phase.

The S phase is the stage of the cell cycle in which the main molecular event of division takes place — DNA replication (copying), that is, the cell genome creates a duplicate of itself. Many chemotherapies are particularly effective against cells in this phase.

DNA replication is a complex molecular process involving many proteins. DNA polymerase enzymes (enzymes are catalyst proteins) are actually responsible for copying the DNA, though dozens of other molecules work to ensure the necessary "working conditions" for these enzymes to do their job. Helicase and topoisomerase proteins help "unwind" the double helix, and SSB proteins bind to single-stranded DNA, preventing it from inevitably getting "tangled up" with complementary strands. The primase protein synthesizes small "primers," which are necessary to ensure that the "main" DNA polymerase can start its job. The ligase enzyme "stitches" the ends of the synthesized DNA fragments, forming a single, continuous strand, etc.

Alkylating drugs (the very same mustard gas derivatives and their analogues we described above) "cross link" DNA molecules and prevent them from dividing. These drugs act on cells at any stage in the cell cycle, but "naked" DNA molecules, which have been freed from their protective proteins and are ready to be copied, are particularly sensitive to them. Much in the same way, cisplatin, the drug mentioned above, "glues" DNA threads and platinum compounds together.

Antimetabolites are another class of drug that have a particularly strong effect on cells in any phase. These are presented as "wrong" or "corrupted" nucleotides that disrupt the synthesis of new DNA, and "corrupted" folic acid analogues that are necessary for purine synthesis (the same antifolates first used by Dr. Farber). This class of drugs includes those such as methotrexate.

Topoisomerase is a protein that "unravels" the DNA double helix during the replication process. Inhibitors of this enzyme also disrupt the division process during the S phase and have an anti-tumor effect. Anthracycline antibiotics are one example.

The S phase is followed by the second preparatory phase, G2, which is followed by a phase of visible cell division (mitosis), known as the M phase. Initially, the cell's nucleus divides into two, and then the cytoplasm is divided between the two new cells. In order for the chromosomes to be evenly distributed between the two daughter cells, the dividing cell's microtubules must form a special structure known as a "division spindle." Drugs that prevent microtubules from assembling, such as anti-tumor drugs known as taxanes, disrupt cell division in this phase.

Healthy cells have special mechanisms to ensure division quality control. In each cell cycle, there are several critical moments or cell cycle control checkpoints, in which the accuracy of the genetic material being copied is checked. If the cell has successfully passed the checkpoint, it will continue to "move" through the cell cycle. Should any circumstances, such as DNA damage, prevent the cell from passing this stage, the cell will either "repair" itself using the DNA repair factors we discussed previously, or die off. The strategic task of chemotherapy is to bring the cancer cells to the "control checkpoints" when they are in their most damaged state — literally bringing them to their death. In order to do this, it is best to affect several processes simultaneously, which is why patients undergoing chemotherapy are often prescribed several drugs from different pharmacological classes at once.

FACT: Classical chemotherapy is aimed at destroying any cells that are actively dividing in the body, while the new generation of drugs attacks tumor cells alone, by taking advantage of specific genetic mutations. This causes less damage to healthy tissues. However, these drugs have not yet been developed for all types of cancer and cannot yet entirely replace chemotherapy.

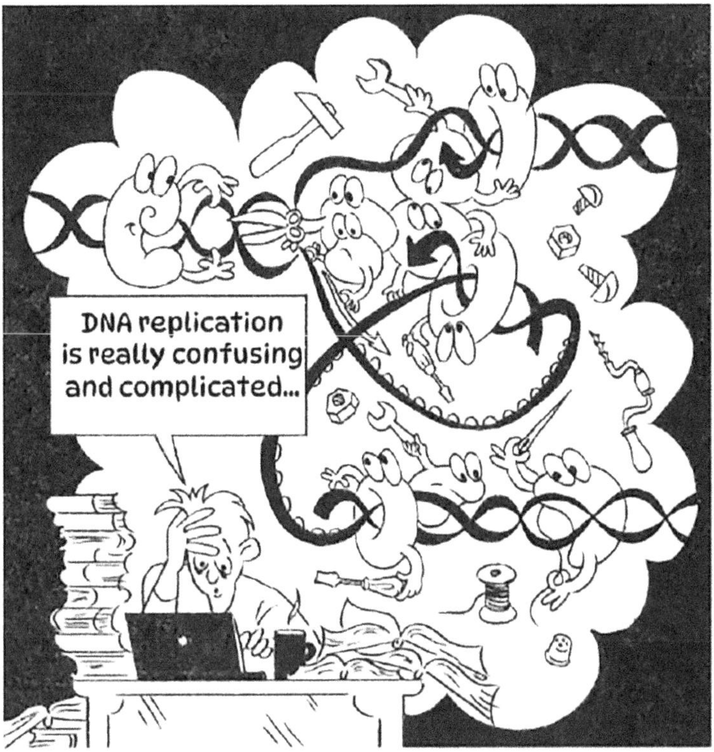

Figure 8. DNA replication (duplication) is a key moment in the cell cycle. The mother's double helix is "unraveled," and the two resulting single strands of DNA are used to create two new DNA helices which will later be divided among the daughter cells. This is a crucial process controlled by a complex set of proteins performing various functions (ligases, helicases, polymerases, etc.).

A VARIETY OF EFFECTIVE THERAPIES

There are already dozens of chemotherapy drugs, with more coming out each year. Why do we need so many drugs if they all work in more or less the same way? Why can we not just pick the most effective and least toxic drugs from what we already have?

Despite the fact that the general principles of cytotoxic chemotherapies are almost identical, for various reasons that are not always well understood, tumors in different locations in the body react differently to the same chemotherapy medications. This is likely related to the fact that though the general cell division mechanisms are universal, at the molecular level the processes taking place in different types of cells are not always the same. As an example, we might look at two different medications based on platinum compounds — cisplatin and oxaliplatin. These drugs have a similar chemical structure and (we assume) act on DNA in more or less the same way. However, cisplatin is a highly effective first-line treatment for testicular cancer (though it is also used for other types of cancers), while oxaliplatin is more effective for treating rectal cancer. Other drugs show similar selectivity.

However, the main problem here (not only when it comes to cytostatics such as those above, but with many other types of cancer treatments) is that, very often, tumors that initially seem to respond to the drug are defeated, only to return later in a form that resists previous treatments. The patient known to us by the initials J. D., who was the first to receive chemotherapy, did live several months longer than doctors had expected, though he eventually died when his lymphosarcoma returned. Dr. Farber's young patients also met the same fate — their rapid remission was followed by an equally rapid relapse, and eventual death. Though these patients were suffering from terminal (at the time) diseases and the pioneering treatment gave them a few extra months of life, researchers were very discouraged by the unstable results of those first clinical trials. The theory of evolution helped researchers to understand why these cancerous tumors seemed to have such astonishing vitality and the ability to resurrect themselves time and again, rising from the ashes like wicked phoenixes.

It appears that most tumors begin with a single precancerous cell, but this cell's offspring will accumulate different mutations at different rates, which means that tumor cells will not only lose their similarity to the original "mother" tissue, but they will also greatly differ among themselves. This internal heterogeneity is a feature of cancer tissue that is very important for understanding how the disease develops. What appears to be a single entity — a tumor — is in fact more of a hydra of like-minded individuals, or a collection of generally "selfish" cells that are using a living organism's limited resources. In line with Darwin's theory about the "survival of the fittest," these cells begin a fight for survival among themselves, in which the most efficient clones will prevail. Alas, the more "efficient" the tumor, the worse the patient's prognosis.

Once a patient begins receiving chemotherapy, the treatment acts like an additional factor of natural selection for the cancer cells. Just as we now see the emergence of antibiotic-resistant bacteria (a problem that is growing more serious with each passing year), when chemotherapy is insufficiently effective, the cancerous tumor will develop a resistance. All it takes is a few cells with the necessary mutations allowing them to survive in a toxic environment for the tumor to relapse. This is why, just as with antibiotics, the treating oncologist will keep other treatment options in mind, in case the patient stops responding. The broader the range of drugs and the greater the possibility to combine them and achieve a stronger (synergistic) response, the higher the patient's chances of beating the cancer will be.

Oncologists had already reached this conclusion during the early days of chemotherapy. None of the first-generation chemotherapy drugs led to a stable remission in leukemia patients, and it was not until these patients were offered a treatment regimen consisting of several drugs capable of hitting various "weak points" in the cell cycle that doctors managed to actually see most patients completely recover. This approach of treating patients with several drugs simultaneously is still used in oncology today, even though some modern drugs are so effective that monotherapy (treatment with just one drug) appears to be sufficient. The second principle of chemotherapy—"bring out the reserves"—was also formulated during this era. This means that the therapy should not be stopped at the first signs of improvement, but rather continued for several weeks, in order to "finish off" the enemy and attempt to leave no chance of survival, even for single tumor cells. Unfortunately, both of these principles — using several drugs at once and continuing the treatment for a longer period of time — will worsen chemo's side effects.

Chemotherapy inherently affects all actively dividing cells in an organism — and this is why it involves so many side effects. The cells of the intestines, hair follicles, and, more importantly, hematopoietic and immune cells renew at a high rate, and are therefore the inevitable casualties of cancer treatments. For this reason, the drugs are usually prescribed in cycles, so the body has a chance to recover. Doctors have learned to mitigate some of chemotherapy's negative side effects, for example, by using special cooling helmets in order to slow down the metabolic processes, reducing the damaging effects of cytotoxic drugs on hair follicles. As a result, patients do not lose as much hair during treatment (this is especially important to female patients). Similar cooling bandages also prevent damage to the fingernails and toenails. This may not seem like a big deal to those of us on the outside, but from the patient's perspective, these small details can greatly affect their self-esteem, the impact of which should not be underestimated when it comes to treatment success.

Sometimes, drugs used in chemotherapy, such as alkylating agents, are themselves mutagenic, and might cure one tumor only to cause another to form. These factors complicate the difficult task of selecting cancer drug therapy, which does not always have one right solution, even with today's range of treatment possibilities.

Unfortunately, as we have already seen, there is no chemotherapy alternative for many types of cancer, though researchers are actively studying new, more-targeted, and less-toxic methods capable of halting actively dividing cancer cells.

FACT: Cancerous tumors are capable of evolving and changing their properties.

Superheroes walk among us

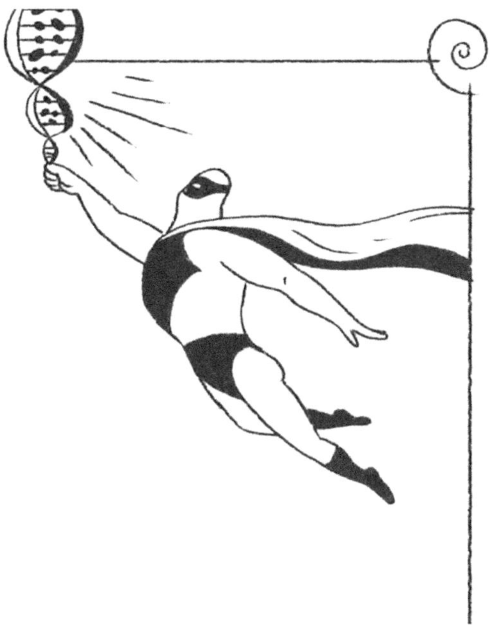

For years, researching the genetic nature of diseases followed a pattern: we would take several (the more, the better) patients with the same clinical picture and scan their genomes, and if we found one or more similar mutations, we would conclude that those mutations were associated with the disease. This is how scientists discovered that cystic fibrosis is caused by a point mutation (really a group of point mutations) in a one-and-only transport protein. This methodology also led to the discovery of the link between the BRCA gene and inherited forms of breast cancer.

However, several years ago, when genome sequencing became more widespread, researchers decided to check whether such mutations only occur in patients with the diseases they cause. The results were stunning. It turns out that there are many people who are out there, walking around and carrying various mutated genes associated with severe genetic diseases, and yet they are alive and well, having blissfully never suffered in the slightest from the disorders caused by their genome. American scientist Stephen Friend only half-jokingly refers to such people as "superheroes," as each of them must have some kind of "superpower" just like the heroes in popular comics, allowing them to neutralize these dangerous mutations. Many laboratories around the world are now busy studying the material nature of this "superpower," and scientists hope that, one day, these compensatory mechanisms working in genetic "superheroes" can be used to help people suffering from various hereditary diseases. For the rest of us, this example serves as a reminder that the "gene–disease" relationship is not quite as straightforward as it may seem.

WHERE SIGNAL PATHWAYS LEAD

A diagram of the cell cycle from one division to the next might look like the wheel on a water mill, but what exactly makes that wheel spin? Why is it that in some cases, the wheel turns smoothly, while in others, it starts whirling like crazy? To answer this question, which is directly linked to modern, targeted cancer therapies, we must remember the ability to interact with one's environment, which is yet another property of living beings.

To live is to react. Obeying signals from the outside, a hungry amoeba will move toward a potential food source or "curl up" as a spore until the situation improves. In more highly organized organisms like (presumably) you and me, those reactions to the outside environment also go hand in hand with social interactions, allowing us to solve complicated tasks that are simply too much for a single individual to handle on their own. We do not just take a warm jacket out of the closet when we learn there is about to be a cold snap or open up the refrigerator when we get hungry. We also exchange information with our colleagues, we make plans with our loved ones, we express approval or disapproval of the actions of those in our social group. However, few of us think about the fact that our own bodies are, in a way, the same kind of society, a union of many different cells that must work in incredible coordination to keep us alive. In order to exchange information with one another, cells use various chemical (molecular) signals. The pathways that these signals use to change cell behavior in one way or another are known as signaling pathways. The most well-known signaling molecules, which everyone has heard of, are hormones. Sex hormones determine the shape of our body (male or female) and our ability to reproduce. Insulin is a hormone that regulates our body's ability to metabolize glucose among other things. All of these hormones (as well as other, less-known mediating molecules) have their own pathways to send messages to a cell.

Most signal molecules (also known as ligands) are proteins or other fairly large molecules that are too big to enter a cell by passing through the membrane. In order to transmit a signal, they must bind to a special receptor protein, which looks like a fish, in that it is embedded in the outer cell membrane so that the "head" is on the outside and the "tail" is inside the cell. When the "head" captures the ligand, the receptor molecule changes its shape, and its intracellular "tail" transmits the signal further.

This is a convenient system, in that by regulating the number of some receptors on their surface, the cells determine what signals they will react to, and which they will ignore. For example, estrogen hormone receptors are mainly present in the cells of the female reproductive organs and mammary glands and are much less present in other tissues. This means that these organs (especially the ovaries and uterus) will react to changes in the level of sex hormones during the menstrual cycle, while others (the liver, stomach, lungs, etc.) will not be affected by this signal.

Hormones are transported fairly evenly throughout the body by blood and other fluids, but it is the particular receptor "repertoire" in each specific cell that determines to which "molecular messages" it will respond. This is more or less the same principle used to arrange emails by topic within a company — some messages only go to the accounting department, others to sales, and yet others are for the entire company.

In healthy tissues, cell division is also subject to signals from the outside, which determine the organism's growth and development as well as its ability to regenerate itself. In cancer cells, however, the set of receptors is different from what is normally present in healthy cells in the same tissue. For example, some receptors, such as those that send a signal restricting cell growth and division, will simply stop being synthesized at all, while others are produced in excess. This change to the molecular repertoire explains the cancer cell's "disobedience" and its ability to "do what it wants," ignoring orders coming from the body.

After the ligand has bound to the receptor, this triggers a sort of molecular intracellular relay race that aims to strengthen the external signal and deliver it to the cell's nucleus. One protein activates two more, which in turn react by becoming the next intermediaries, which pass the molecular baton on further, involving more and more molecules. Thanks to this signal amplification effect, even tiny doses of hormones (by chemical standards) are capable of causing significant changes in the organism. In the end, this signaling cascade will activate special proteins known as transcription factors, which are able to selectively bind to DNA and activate or block (inhibit) the functions of certain genes. Often, there is a single transcription factor controlling an entire group of genes involved in a specific process. This ensures consistency when synthesizing several protein molecules simultaneously. As a result of changes in the expression level in a group of genes, the cell's "protein repertoire" changes, as do the functions it performs. This is how an adequate cellular response to an external signal is formed.

The sequence of molecular interactions that begins with the ligand binding and ends with a cellular response (usually the synthesis of certain proteins) is called a signaling cascade or signaling pathway. In this book, we are mainly focused on the signaling pathways related to cell cycle regulation, but the general principles of transmitting signals described above are the same for all of the body's major cellular processes. The immune response and programmed cell death mechanisms, which play a major role in cancer, have their own signaling pathways, which we will discuss below.

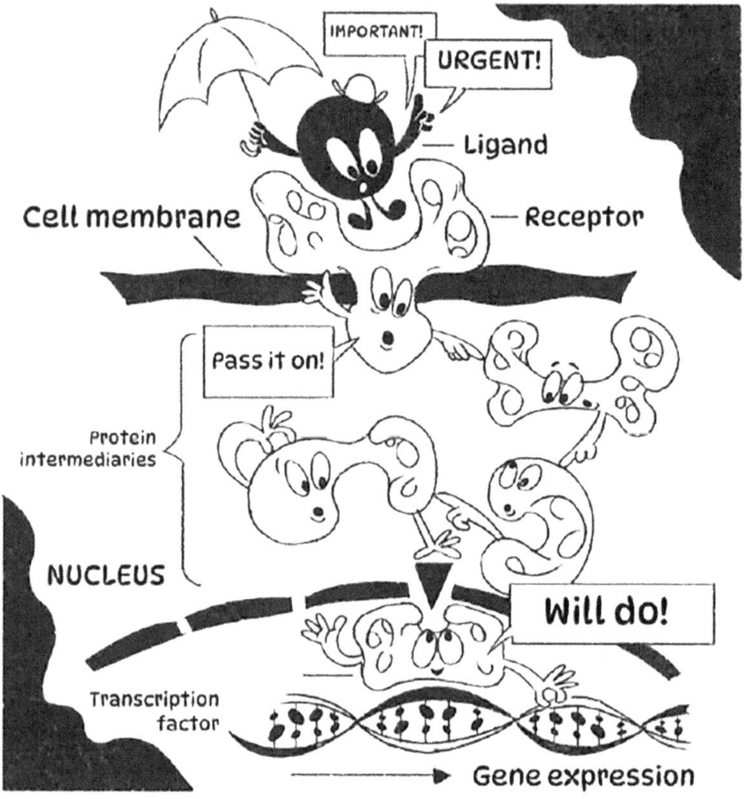

Figure 9. Signaling pathways make it possible to regulate intracellular processes in response to external signals. Molecular messengers, or ligands, will bind to receptor proteins on the cell's surface, triggering a reaction cascade, which causes changes in the activities of certain genes.

Rather than a living cell, imagine any factory, for example, a cell phone assembly line. There are workers on the line, but the supervisor standing at the machine is not the person who decides how many gadgets need to be produced each day. That decision comes from a long management chain. First, the marketing department receives information on sales (a signal from the outside). This is put into a report sent to factory management (transmitting the signal from the outside to the inside of the cell). Management then sends instructions to increase the production of a certain kind of model to the secretary, who turns it into an internal order and sends it to the shop floor (intracellular signal transmission), and only then will the supervisors start their machines.

If we leave the industrial metaphors behind and come back to biological processes, it is important to understand that the "machines" on the molecular conveyor belt associated with cellular division, such as proteins that ensure the synthesis of DNA molecules and control the assembly and divergence of chromosomes, are very rarely damaged in cancer. The mutations that disrupt the function of these key macromolecules are usually lethal — they lead to cell death. An error that causes malignant transformation is usually in the "plant management," or upstream part of the signaling pathway. It is the cellular division regulation, rather than the division itself, that is disrupted.

Here is one more "technical" metaphor to help us visualize the drama of what is happening. A cancer cell looks like a car with an engine that works perfectly, but the brakes stick, and the steering wheel is jammed — it is fast and out of control.

After the previous chapter, we already know that mutations in the genes that code two groups of proteins — oncogenes and oncosuppressors — are critical for tumor development. If we analyze their biochemical features, among them we will find molecules with several different functions — receptors, enzymes, and transcription factors, among others. At first glance, they seem to have nothing in common! But if we look closely, it turns out that all of these proteins are either directly or indirectly involved in the signaling pathways that regulate cell growth and division.

FACT: Cancer is a genetic disease that causes a disruption in the cell cycle regulation processes, and therefore results in increased cell division.

TREATING THE SIGNALING PATHWAYS, BOTH INSIDE AND OUT

The main ligands that trigger the cell cycle in the human body are a group of proteins called growth factors (GF). Their name usually includes a reference to the tissue in which their effect was first or most clearly described — epidermal growth factor, hepatocyte growth factor, etc. Each of these GFs acts through its specific receptors (or group of receptors). By sending a signal to the cell nucleus via a chain of intermediaries, the GFs trigger the synthesis of special proteins known as cyclins.

Cyclins are the cell cycle's main regulators. A graph of changes in the levels of various cyclins in a cell looks like a drawing of waves overlapping one another, each bringing the cell to the next phase of division. In turn, cyclins activate special enzymes — cyclin-dependent kinases (CDKs) and others, right up to proteins that directly regulate DNA copying and chromosome divergence. The 2001 Nobel Prize went to scientists Leland Hartwell, Timothy Hunt, and Paul Nurse, for explaining the mechanisms of cell cycle regulation by cyclins and CDKs.

A detailed description of the signaling pathways leading to cell division is worthy of an entire book in itself, but in order to understand the general principles of malignant transformation, there are a few basic points we can understand. A genetic disorder can affect the signaling pathway that leads to cell division at many different levels of regulation. A cell can start intensively producing GFs or GF receptors, or the cyclin mechanisms or transcription factor regulation can be broken, etc. But the end result will be the same — an amplification of molecular signals telling the cell: "Divide!" As we mentioned earlier, oncogenes and oncosuppressors can be a variety of different proteins along the signaling cascade that triggers cell division. For example, the well-known oncogene called MYC is a transcription factor, as is oncosuppressor p53, and oncogenic RAS proteins are enzymes. These "molecular details" are invisible to the naked eye, but extremely important in terms of developing and applying targeted drug therapy that is not aimed at all dividing cells (like traditional chemotherapy), but only at those carrying a specific genetic breakdown.

Mutations associated with molecules on the cell's surface or in the extracellular environment are easier to compensate for with drugs than intracellular signaling disorders. Ligands and receptors are more accessible for interventions than cyclins or CDKs. After all, in order to reach cyclins or CDKs, the drugs need to cross the cell membrane barrier, which is not a simple task. This is why today, cancers in which pathological cell division is associated with excessive activity in certain receptors (usually as a result of amplification, or an increase in the number of copies of their genes) have seen the greatest success with treatment from targeted therapy.

One classic example of this type of oncogenic receptor is the *HER2* protein. Increased synthesis of this protein is present in 20–30 percent of breast cancer patients, which causes accelerated tumor growth. Trastuzumab (also known as Herceptin) is a drug based on antibodies to this receptor. On one hand, it blocks the GF signal and stops cell division in the tumor, and on the other, it attracts immune system cells. (In normal conditions, an organism's antibodies "tag" any "foreign" cells, such as bacteria, but we will discuss this in greater detail in the chapter on cancer immunotherapies.) The immune cells recognize the antibodies on the surface of the cells that are overproducing *HER2* and destroy them.

Sex hormones are a separate and very important group of ligands that accelerate cell division. The signaling pathways associated with these molecules are mostly active in the sex organs. Disruptions in the signaling pathways for the hormones progesterone and estrogen can lead to the development of female tumors, such as some types of breast, uterine, and ovarian cancers. Prostate cancer is the most common type of male tumor that is sensitive to testosterone levels. As with

GFs, the general principle for treating hormone-dependent tumors is based on blocking (inhibiting) hormone signals at some stage. This type of treatment is known as "hormone" therapy, though "anti-hormone" therapy would probably be a more accurate term.

During the development of this treatment method, it became clear that male sex hormones in the female body work differently than female sex hormones in the male body. The introduction of high levels of female sex hormone analogues (synthetic estrogen, or diethylstilbestrol) into a man's body will almost entirely block the synthesis of the male hormone testosterone by inhibiting the normal signal from the pituitary gland to the testes, halting the development of prostate cancer. This method of "chemical castration" was widely used for the treatment of hormone-dependent tumors in men during the 1960s, until it was replaced by safer methods of regulating patients' hormonal status. American physiologist Charles Huggins won the 1966 Nobel Prize for developing a hormonal treatment for malignant prostate tumors.

During the hormonal treatment of prostate cancer, patients will begin to show signs of "feminization"—weight gain and loss of body hair, for example — but these changes are reversible and will go away once the course of treatment has been completed. Nonetheless, the introduction of high doses of testosterone in female breast cancer patients led to many side effects related to "masculinization" (increased body hair, deepening of the voice), but did not have a noticeable effect on their tumors. Instead, researchers had to approach female-hormone-dependent cancers from the other direction, synthesizing substances capable of blocking the receptors for these hormones.

There is an interesting story related to the advent of one of the most common drugs for estrogen-dependent breast cancer — tamoxifen. Initially, the molecule was tested as a potential contraceptive, but did not show satisfactory results. However, its ability to reliably block estrogen receptors made it an effective treatment for estrogen-sensitive female tumors.

As with any targeted therapy, hormonal cancer therapy requires an understanding of the molecular features of the patient's specific tumor. (It makes no sense to give tamoxifen to a patient if her tumor does not express estrogen receptors.) This type of therapy will only be prescribed once a detailed genetic and biochemical analysis of the tumor has been completed.

Though reaching intracellular oncogenes is much more difficult than turning a receptor on the membrane surface "on" or "off," there have been some successes in this area as well. One example of such a drug has been imatinib (Glivec), a targeted drug for treating one type of "blood cancer"—chronic myeloid leukemia. This disease is characterized by a specific chromosomal arrangement, which results in the "head" of chromosome 22 and the "tail" of chromosome 9 merging to form the so-called Philadelphia chromosome. This leads to a hybrid gene (and hybrid protein) *BCR-ABL*, which leads to the pathological division of blood cells. From a biochemical point of view, the *BCR-ABL* protein (along with many other oncogenes) is a "frantic" and hyperactive kinase, which indiscriminately and uncontrollably phosphorylates cell cycle proteins. The active ingredient in imatinib is a complex organic molecule (not a protein!) capable of selectively binding to a "molecular pocket" on the surface of this hybrid kinase and completely blocking its activity. Thanks to imatinib, chronic myeloid leukemia, which was once an almost incurable disease, is now a cancer with a nearly 100 percent recovery rate.

FACT: Targeted therapy today mainly aims at ligands and receptors (not only in cancer cells), but in some cases, it is also possible to achieve a targeted effect on proteins acting inside the cell.

HUMANS AND DISEASE

In writing this book, I most wanted to write about the cellular and molecular nature of cancer, but of course that is an impossible task without remembering that each drug has traveled a long, difficult path from its initial conception in the laboratory to its official release on the pharmaceutical market, and there is a story of human hope and desperation, lives saved, and, sadly, lives lost as well.

The dramatic story of the first clinical trial of the *HER2* receptor–specific drug trastuzumab we read about earlier in this chapter was described by American physician Siddhartha Mukherjee in his book *The Emperor of All Maladies: A Biography of Cancer*. Here he describes the experience of one patient, Barbara Bradfield:

The lump on Bradfield's neck — the only tumor in the group that could be physically touched, measured, and watched — became the compass for the trial. On the morning of the first intravenous infusion of the Her-2 antibody, all the women came up to feel the lump, one by one, running their hands across Bradfield's collarbone. It was a peculiarly intimate ritual that would be repeated every week. Two weeks after the first dose of the antibody, when the group filed past Bradfield, touching the node again, the change was incontrovertible. Bradfield's tumor had softened and visibly shrunk. "We began to believe that something was happening here," Bradfield recalled. "Suddenly, the weight of our good fortune hit us."

Not everyone was as fortunate as Bradfield. Exhausted and nauseous one evening, a young woman with relapsed metastatic cancer was unable to keep down the fluids needed to hydrate her body. She vomited through the night and then, too tired to keep drinking and too sick to understand the consequences, fell back into sleep. She died of kidney failure the next week.

Barbara was truly lucky. Her tumor, which was literally "swollen" by the extra copies of the *HER2* gene, completely disappeared thanks to the therapy. Barbara Bradfield completed her treatment in 1993, and by the time Mukherjee's book was published in 2006, she was in good health. But the dramatic story of the new drug trial does not end there. The procedure for licensing new drugs was very complicated, lengthy, and highly bureaucratic in the 1990s. The company Genentech (which owned the development) had to carry out many clinical trials before it could officially launch the drug on the market. Meanwhile, the news of a new, effective drug was spreading like wildfire among breast cancer patients. Many of those patients, especially those in whom the cancer had already begun to spread throughout their bodies, as in the case of Barbara Bradfield, were willing to take a chance on trying an experimental drug, as they saw it as their last chance at recovery. However, due to the regulations in place, Genentech was prevented from providing these patients with the drug, and insurance companies were prevented from paying for the expensive, experimental treatment. The conflict between the pharmaceutical company and government oversight services reached its pinnacle with the story of Marti Nelson. For a long time, Nelson's insurance company had refused to approve testing her tumor for *HER2* expression, and without the test, Genentech would not provide her with the drug. As a result of the head-butting between the two entities, a very young, forty-one-year-old woman died of a rapidly progressing cancer that probably could have been stopped.

After Nelson's death, the conflict between patients and Genentech turned into direct confrontation. In December 1994, a crowd of breast-cancer-patient rights activists stormed the Genentech company campus with signs depicting Marti Nelson shortly before her death. A wave of public outrage forced the company to reconsider its policies, and as a result, patients gained access to experimental drugs, and patient organizations became recognized as a political (and economic) force capable of influencing clinical research.

FACT: Chemotherapy helps many people but will not save everyone. No one cancer treatment can pro vide a 100 percent guarantee of recovery. However, the same could also be said about many other diseases, including something as “ordinary” as pneumonia. Today’s medicine is powerful, but not all-powerful.

SUMMARY

In this chapter, we learned how classical chemotherapy and modern, targeted therapies kill cancer cells by interfering with cell division.

We learned about the basic cellular processes that determine the life cycle of a cell, from one division to the next, and we saw that most oncogenes and oncosuppressors are fragments of the signaling pathways that regulate cell division. This knowledge has allowed researchers and physicians to shift from developing general cytostatic drugs that affect all dividing cells to searching for a new generation of drugs that act on specific molecules, causing damage to a particular tumor, through a signaling cascade.

This has been a long and winding path of both victories and defeats. While it was rather easy to neutralize the harmful effect of excessive synthesis of ligands and receptors that activate cell division, repressing oncogenes within the cell (such as the KRAS protein) has proven to be a much more difficult task. However, scientists continue to research in this area, and there is no doubt that the number of "targeted" therapies that stop the division of cancer cells will grow in the coming years and, in time, they will at least displace traditional chemotherapy, if they do not completely supplant it.

In the meantime, there are new questions. There are healthy tissues in our bodies that divide at nearly the same speed as malignant tissues, and which also suffer from chemotherapy — for example, the intestinal mucosa or hair follicles. But these tissues do not form tumors, so does that mean that cancer is not just about cellular reproduction? If that is the case, then what is it? In the next chapter, we will discuss how growth, development, and death are balanced in a healthy body, and how a tumor disrupts that process.

Chapter 4.
THE STORY OF HeLa AND MYTHS ABOUT DEATH AND IMMORTALITY

A malignant tumor holds secrets that both terrify us and excite our wildest imaginations. The dream of eternal life is probably humankind's oldest hope, as we can guess based on so many myths and legends.

Cancer cells are immortal — at least, that is what people claim. But what if we could learn immortality from them? Headlines like "Can Cancer Give Us Immortality?" pop up with alarming frequency in supposedly "scientific" news feeds. Is that the case? The correct answer to this question is complicated. The study of cancer cells and the use of tumor cell lines such as HeLa are progressing in many areas of biological science, including the science of aging (gerontology), so the answer is at least partly "yes." But it is simply impossible to borrow molecular strategies of immortality from tumor cells and apply them to such a complex multicellular organism as a human being, so the rest of the answer is a resounding "no."

In order to understand what is true and what is false in this widespread notion of cancer cells' immortality and its relationship to prospects for extending the human lifespan, we will need to carefully study the molecular mechanisms of programmed cell death, or apoptosis; learn how tumor tissues are so similar yet so different from embryonic tissue; and also understand why stem cells, which are responsible for renewing our bodies, are also the culprit behind some tumors.

WHEN DEATH IS A BLESSING

Ancient Greek philosopher Heraclitus wrote, "People do not understand how what is borne in different directions comes to be in agreement with itself; [for] a framework like that of the bow and the lyre turns back [on itself]," meaning that life and death are inseparable. No matter how tragic the passing of each individual human being and even some beloved animals may be, on a global biosphere level, our mortality is what makes life as a whole possible. Without a balance between reproduction and extinction, living matter would soon cease to exist, having rapidly depleted the resources it needs. Religions such as Christianity promise "eternal life" with a "new heaven" and "new earth," but without this additional assumption, a paradise populated by immortal, still-hungry and still-reproducing creatures would quickly descend into hell.

Without the mortality of individual organisms, there is no evolution, no development, and no selectivity — the essential qualities of life. Philosopher-economist Nassim Taleb writes about this in his book *Antifragile:*[4]

To satisfy the conditions for such immortality, the organisms need to predict the future with perfection — near perfection is not enough. But by letting the organisms go one lifespan at a time, with modifications between successive generations, nature does not need to predict future conditions beyond the extremely vague idea of which direction things should be heading. Actually, even a vague direction is not necessary. Every random event will bring its own antidote in the form of ecological variation. It is as if nature changed itself at every step and modified its strategy every instant.

---

[4] Nassim Taleb, Antifragile: Things That Gain from Disorder (New York: Random House, 2012).

In order for *Homo sapiens* as we know them to have formed, several dozen less fortunate species of hominids had to die out. Perhaps humanity will eventually achieve immortality, but the very fact that our species came into existence thanks to natural selection (that is, biological death) of other life forms will not be undone. We should be grateful for death — and for life. At first glance, that may seem like a paradoxical statement.

The human body, like any multicellular organism, is a complex union of different cells subject to a common genetic program. Maintaining our health and genetic integrity involves constant renewal — the death of some cells and the division of others.

If human cells only divided and never died, then the human body would continue growing in size throughout our lifespan, eventually reaching enormous and unviable dimensions. Boris Zhivotovsky, an expert on programmed cell death, often cites the example of frequently dividing intestinal cells in his lectures. If old cells did not die, by the age of seventy, this key organ would have grown to nearly forty kilometers in length.

In contrast, if human body cells stopped dividing entirely once we reached adulthood, those that are constantly being exposed to harmful factors (for example, the cells of the skin or digestive system), would accumulate mutations at such a rate that they would quickly lose their ability to perform their functions. This is to say nothing of the fact that the body would lose its ability to heal from even a minor scratch (regeneration requires accelerated cell division).

Fortunately, our body does have mechanisms to maintain a balance between cell death and cell division. This allows our body to efficiently shed cells that have accumulated a "critical mass" of genetic errors, and remove the burden of somatic mutations. Prolonging the human lifespan seems like an increasingly achievable goal, but we need to keep in mind that an immortal human body as a whole would never involve the immortality of each individual cell.

This is also true for tumors. Individual cancer cells are not immortal by any stretch. Even in the absence of treatment, the individual cells that make up the neoplasm die en masse due to an accumulation of too many genetic errors or a lack of oxygen (hypoxia). However, because, in general, division processes predominate cell death processes, the tumor will continue to exist and grow.

FACT: Both division and natural death regulation processes are disrupted in cancerous tumors. This means that malignant neoplasms can survive with genetic errors that would usually be lethal to healthy cells.

APOPTOSIS – DYING TO LIVE

The word apoptosis means "falling leaf" in Greek, a rather poetic description of dying off and renewal. Old leaves fall off to make way for fresh, green shoots. Old cells do the same, dying off and allowing new tissues and the organism as a whole to be renewed. However, the purpose of apoptosis is not limited to the mechanical process of replacing the old with the new.

Research on programmed cell death began in the 1960s, and scientists quickly understood that apoptosis is one of the key processes guiding the development of any multicellular organism (in 2002, Sydney Brenner, Robert Horvitz, and John Sulston won the Nobel Prize in Physiology or Medicine for their research on the role of apoptosis in living organisms).

When Michelangelo was asked about how he began a sculpture, he answered, "I just take the stone and cut off everything unnecessary." Apoptosis in a developing organism is like a chisel in a sculptor's hands. The most well-known example of this, which is something every school child has seen in science class, is the disappearance of a tadpole's tail as it grows into a frog.

In much the same way, "trimming the fat" is part of the development of the human embryo. You probably know that at a certain stage, all of us have a tail, gills, and webbing between our fingers. Perhaps, when looking at images describing the stages of development in the human embryo, you wondered where all of these features go as the fetus develops. Now, we know: these archaic structures are removed through apoptosis during embryogenesis, giving way to new and more progressive forms. As genetic experiments on lab animals have shown, embryos with abnormalities in the genes that regulate this process die during the early stages of embryogenesis from intractable developmental defects. In adult organisms, apoptosis mainly serves to maintain cellular homeostasis — keeping the cell population at the same quantity and quality.

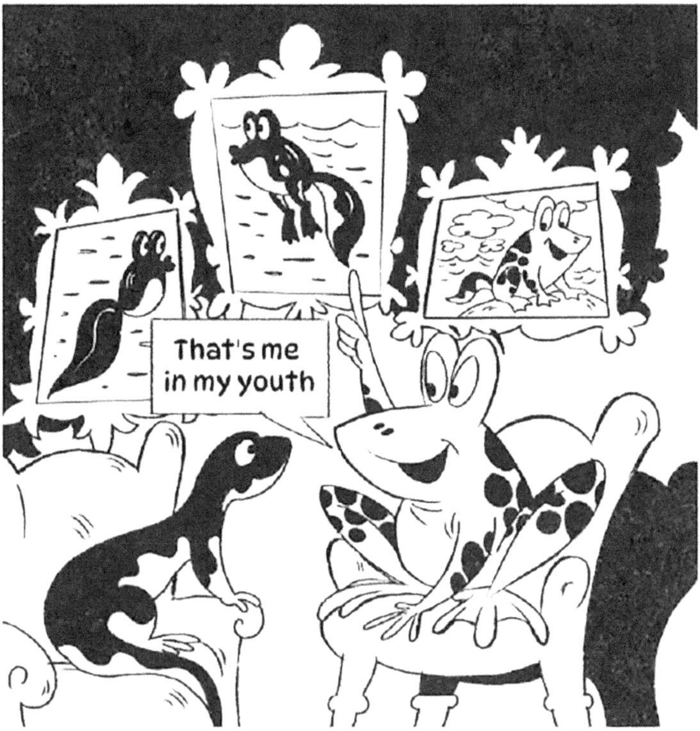

Figure 10. Apoptosis "dissolves" the growing tadpole's tail as it transforms into a frog.

In school, we all studied biology and learned about the ecological relationship between predators and prey, and that wolves act as "game wardens" for deer and elk, first hunting the weaker and sicker animals, and preventing the healthier ones from reproducing too much and depleting the food supply. In a healthy organism, apoptosis acts like the wolf when it comes to weak, sick, and simply excessive cells. The only difference is that death does not come from the outside, but from within. This way, apoptosis is more like hara-kiri, or ritual suicide committed by a loyal Japanese samurai warrior, who has realized that he is no longer useful to his master.

The total mass of cells in our organism that self-destruct each year is approximately the same weight as a full-grown adult human. In a way, we are indeed reborn every year!

How does this cellular hara-kiri take place? The cytoplasm of any cell has inactive caspase proteins, which are similar to the enzymes in our digestive tract that break down proteins and nucleic acids that we ingest as food. During apoptosis, these enzymes activate and "digest" the contents of the cell. The process is quick and sudden — the cell membrane begins to bubble, and the entire cytoplasm seems to boil over. Scientists very poetically refer to this as the "dance of death," a reference to a popular medieval European painting.

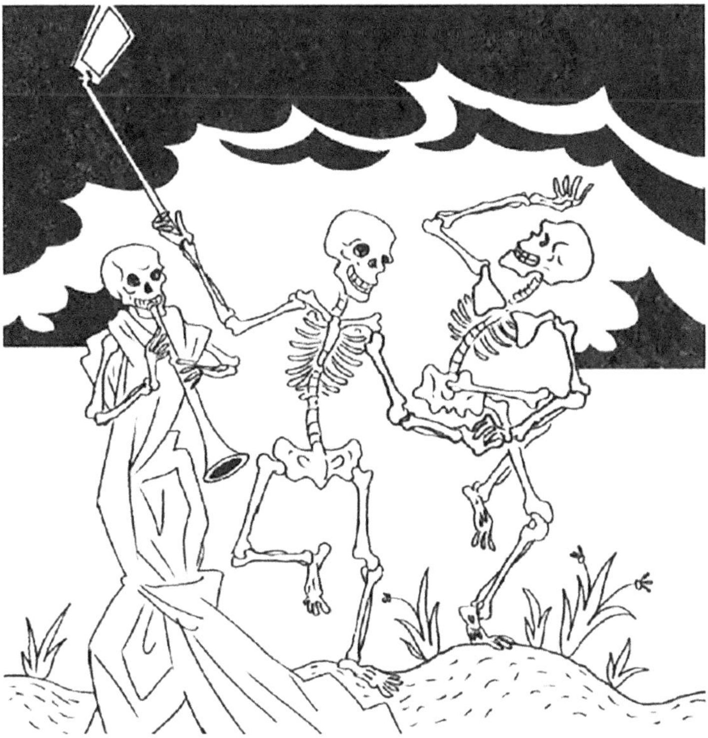

Figure 11. "The dance of death"—scientists compare the way that cells frantically "boil" during apoptosis to the subjects of this medieval engraving. In cancer cases, the regulation of this process is disrupted, one of the key signs of malignant transformation (see Figure 1).

However, unlike traumatic or infectious cell damage, when the entire cell contents simply "fall out," causing an inflammatory reaction, normal apoptosis is a very careful process. Splitting the cellular proteins and amino acids does not disturb the integrity of the lipid membrane. In the end, once they have "danced enough," the cellular "broth" is neatly packed into a so-called apoptotic body, which is quickly "eaten" by the immune system, which operates on the principle of "waste nothing you can use." Soon, the space that has just been cleared is occupied by a new, freshly divided cell.

Apoptosis is not the only method for regulating cell death that we know of today. There are also autophagy, necrosis, ferroptosis, and others. In all, scientists currently know of over a dozen processes for cell death. Biologists are actively studying their roles in both normal and pathological processes.

FACT: The mechanisms for regulated cell death, of which apoptosis is the best known, are as inherent to our biological nature as cellular division.

ONCOLOGY'S "STAR MOLECULE"—P53

In the previous chapter on cell division, we talked about cell cycle "checkpoints" during which the cell will check the quality of the genome copying and whether or not it contains any errors. If there are too many errors, the cell cycle will stop, and the cell is directed toward a programmed cell death. This is a natural way to prevent the reproduction of mutated cells while maintaining the organism's genetic homogeneity. In cancer, this crucial mechanism is usually disrupted, which allows for cancer cells to turn a blind eye to even significant rearrangements of the genome, continuing to divide, and accumulating mutations with each generation.

In many cases, this effect can be associated with damage to a single protein known as p53, which we can rightfully refer to as the "star" of molecular oncology, thanks to the number of studies and publications that have been devoted to it. This is the protein that connects the systems regulating genome stability and apoptosis. Its name harks back to the image of Marvel comic book superheroes. In fact, p53 is the "guardian of the genome," which sounds almost as impressive as "guardian of the galaxy."

There is a famous story about a little boy who had not yet begun to speak by the age of five. Everyone thought he was unable to speak, until one day he yelled, "The soup is burning!" When his parents asked why he had not begun to speak before, he said, "Everything was fine before." The p53 protein is like this little boy. In a normal, healthy cell, this protein is in a bound (inactive) state with MDM2 protein; that is, it is "silent." However, once the body suffers any damage, for example, when ultraviolet radiation causes DNA damage, the MDM2/p53 complex falls apart and the "guardian of the genome" gets to work. This reaction happens in response to various types of cellular stress, from radioactivity to hypoxia (caused by oxygen deficiency), giving a universal, "one-size-fits-all" cellular response.

Initially, an increase in the level of free p53 will trigger a DNA repair mechanism, which should fix any errors in the genome. If this is successful, the protein will stop being released, and its levels will again drop rapidly, as cell life returns to normal. However, if this disruption goes too far, the concentration of p53 in the cell will continue to rise, triggering apoptosis. Thus, the future of the cell once it reaches the "checkpoint"—whether it will continue the cell cycle or die off — is largely dependent on this single protein.

Apoptosis is mainly triggered two ways: from inside the cell (by destroying the mitochondria) and externally (by activating the so-called death receptors). Both methods are regulated by p53. It is a transcription factor protein, which means that it can bind to DNA and regulate the activity of different genes. In human cells, p53 simultaneously triggers the synthesis of one of the FAS death receptors and produces BAX protein, which will destroy the mitochondria when embedded in the membrane of these organelles.

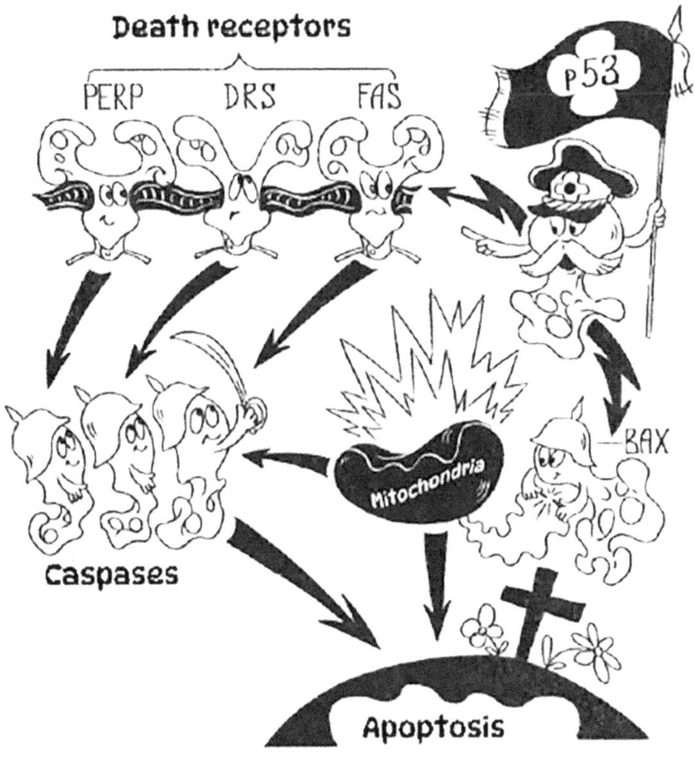

Figure 12. Both main pathways to cellular apoptosis are regulated by p53-externally, from death receptors, and internally, which is related to the destruction of the mitochondria.

When there is a mutation in the *TP53* gene, the corresponding protein's function is impaired. Statistically, 50 to 70 percent of malignant tumors have one or more mutations in the *TP53* gene. As a result, apoptosis regulation is disrupted. Might this be the universal molecule capable of conquering cancer? Maybe the two copies of the *TP53* gene that are present in our bodies are simply not enough to effectively fight the disease, and if, for example, there were four of them and they were more active, would the problem solve itself? Researchers decided to test this assumption and designed genetically modified mice with higher *TP53* gene activity. Compared to their "natural" counterparts, the modified mice did indeed demonstrate remarkable resistance to the formation of malignant tumors. However, they also showed signs of premature aging — vascular disorders, weight loss, etc. Generally speaking, as we often see in biology, it turns out that too much of a good thing is a curse.

What is more, we know that elephants, despite their huge size and a lifespan comparable to that of humans, very rarely get cancer. They also have an increased amount of the *TP53* gene. Genome studies have shown that African elephants have forty copies of *TP53*, while Asian elephants have from thirty to forty. The question whether humans are with the mice or the elephants remains unanswered.

For now, researchers are looking for ways to restore normal *TP53* activity in malignant cells. This is no easy task, because it requires the delivery of a therapeutic agent to the tumor as well as penetrating the cells through the cytoplasmic membrane. (The matter of how to deliver drugs to a specific organ or group of cells is the great bottleneck of modern pharmacology, which tends to wreak havoc on the entire body.)

In order to boost *TP53* activity in cancer cells, researchers use gene therapy methods (when normal *TP53* is delivered to the tumor via an adenoviral vector — an engineered virus) and also search for molecules capable of compensating for defects in the mutated protein. The idea is to find a sort of "molecular crutch" that would allow the p53 protein to function normally within the cell despite the mutation disrupting its structure. The results of this research have not yet reached the clinical trial stage, but the trends look very promising.

Elephant proteins offer one potential path toward treatment for cancerous tumors with damaged p53 proteins. It turns out that elephants have more *TP53* genes than humans, but that the genes they have are far more active in inducing apoptosis than those of their human counterparts. If microcapsules can be created with the capacity of delivering elephant proteins directly to cancer cells, it might present a treatment breakthrough in treating *TP53*-dependent tumors. Given the prevalence of these mutations in cancer, this type of drug might help many patients. Of course, no one would start slaughtering elephants for this purpose. Modern biotechnology methods make it possible to synthesize elephant proteins *in vitro* without harming any of these beautiful and endangered animals.

Disrupting *TP53* gene activity is not the only way that cancer cells can avoid self-destruction. They can also inhibit apoptosis in tumors by speeding up BCL2 activity. The BCL2 protein is a protein antagonist that causes apoptosis by destroying mitochondria. It binds to molecules like the BAK and the BAX we mentioned earlier, blocking their ability to cause apoptosis. Researchers synthesized peptides (short fragments) of these proteins (BH3 mimetics). The peptides adhere to the surface of the BCL2 molecules, reducing their ability to bind to other proteins, and apoptosis is again possible within the cells. Drugs based on BH3 mimetics have been used successfully to treat types of leukemia characterized by increased BCL2 proteins.

By studying apoptosis regulation in cancer cells, scientists have begun to understand the mechanisms of action behind traditional chemotherapy and radiotherapy. It turns out that the mass destruction of DNA by chemical agents or under the influence of radiation leads to the activation of programmed cell death in cancer cells, which multiplies the effect of cytotoxic drugs. Unfortunately, in the case of a *TP53* mutation, that effect stops working, which in part explains why different types of tumors have different sensitivities to chemotherapy.

FACT: A generative mutation in the TP53 gene, which comes from a sperm or egg cell and will eventually be present in all of the body's cells, leads to the development of a rare genetic disease, known as Li-Fraumeni syndrome. This pathological condition, which usually leads to an early death, is characterized in part by the occurrence of multiple tumors in different organs.

TELOMERES – THE BODY'S BUILT-IN AGING SYSTEM

In addition to apoptosis, or rather, along with it, there is another mechanism limiting cell reproduction and the accumulation of mutations in the body — telomere shortening.

In 1961, while studying cellular division, American scientist Leonard Hayflick conducted a simple but very elegant experiment. In a cell culture, he mixed equal amounts of male and female fibroblasts, which were differentiated by the number of cell divisions they had undergone. The male fibroblasts used for the experiment had undergone about forty divisions, while the female cells had undergone about ten (cells of different sexes were used in order to easily differentiate them in the mixture by the presence or absence of the Y chromosome).

At the same time, a control experiment was carried out using the same "old" male fibroblasts, but without adding any female cells. After about ten cell cycles, the control unmixed population of male cells had stopped dividing, while the mixed, experimental culture only contained female cells, as the male cells had all died. Based on these results, Hayflick concluded that normal cells, unlike cancer cells, have a limited ability to divide. This "division limit" later came to be known as the "Hayflick limit." The number of possible divisions differs between different types of cells in the body, but in general falls within the range of forty to sixty divisions. Once the Hayflick limit has been reached, a normal cell will either die or continue working within the body, but no longer enters the cell cycle, remaining in the G0 phase so that any somatic mutations it has managed to accumulate during this time (and continues to accumulate) will stop spreading in the body.

The molecular mechanism explaining the limited number of cellular divisions in normal, mature cells was first theoretically predicted by Soviet scientist Alexey Olovnikov in 1973.

Basically, because human DNA has a linear (chromosome) rather than circular shape, for example, as is the case with bacteria, in each copying cycle, one of the ends will not be fully reproduced. The large protein complex of DNA polymerase enzymes, which ensures that DNA is copied, requires a rather extensive "launch pad" where it lands before beginning its work. This is the same DNA polymerase landing spot on the end of the chromosome that will remain under-copied, each time. After several cycles, the cell's chromosomes gradually become shorter. Olovnikov predicted that after reaching a certain (critical) length, the division process would become impossible, though all other cell functions might be preserved.

Later on, experimental work brilliantly confirmed this hypothesis, and in 2009 American researchers Elizabeth Blackburn, Carol Greider, and Jack Szostak won the Nobel Prize for their study of telomeres and their links to aging (both cell lines and the body as a whole). It turns out that telomere length is a very sensitive and accurate "sensor" as to the state of the individual cells and the body in general, as it responds to stress. Elizabeth Blackburn's laboratory even patented a test to determine a person's biological age (which can be quite different from the one listed on their driver's license) based on the length of their telomeres. However, telomere function in division does not only serve to ensure DNA polymerase landing. This is a special structure which prevents chromosomes from "sticking together" and ensures that they are properly separated during division.

At least — that is how things work in normal, healthy cells. But what happens in cancer cells? It turns out that telomeres retain their "youthful" length and are constantly being renewed, despite the high number of divisions. Special proteins are responsible for renewing telomeres in the cell. The telomerase enzyme, the best known of these, is usually absent in mature cells in an adult's body, but in a tumor cell it is synthesized in large quantities. For many tumors, there is a very unfortunate pattern — the higher the telomerase activity, the worse the patient's prognosis for recovery is. This means that telomerase is an important potential target for drug interventions, and many pharmaceutical companies are currently studying drugs that block telomere elongation.

This is not an easy task: in recent years, research has shown that, as is the case with DNA repair systems, there are multiple systems for telomere elongation (telomerase) working in cancer cells. However, early experimentation has shown that by preventing telomere elongation, it is possible to block the reproduction of many types of cancer cells, including glioblastoma — a brain cancer that does not respond well to most traditional types of chemotherapy. Researchers are leaving no stone unturned when it comes to attempts at controlling this process.

Telomerase is one of many examples of adult cancer cells activating genes that are usually only active in embryos. There is a whole group of cancer markers (proteins that when present can usually be used to predict the presence of a malignant tumor in the body) known as "oncofetal antigens." These are molecules that are normally only produced in human embryonic tissue, and disappear once the fetus is formed. In the case of malignant tumors, however, they begin to be synthesized again, which is why they can be used as markers to diagnose the disease. One of these oncofetal antigens is alpha-fetoprotein, a marker for hepatocellular carcinoma, a type of liver cancer. Soviet researchers G. Abelev and Y. Tatarinov played an important role in the discovery and study of this protein, when they developed an effective method for detecting this tumor marker in blood serum (the Abelev–Tatarinov reaction, or the alpha-fetoprotein test). Another example is carcinoembryonic antigen, a marker for colon cancer. Later on, we will discuss the mechanisms that allow tumor cells to "look so young" at the molecular level.

FACT: One of the most reliable cancer markers today is prostate-specific antigen. High levels of this protein in the blood give physicians reason to suspect early-stage prostate cancer, when the disease is still asymptomatic. For this reason, in many countries, including in Russia, this annual test is recommended for men over the age of forty-five. The American Cancer Society recommends this test beginning at age fifty for men of average risk for prostate cancer, at age forty-five for men at high risk (African Americans and men with a first-degree relative diagnosed with prostate cancer before the age of sixty-five), and at age forty for men at even higher risk.

The story of HeLa

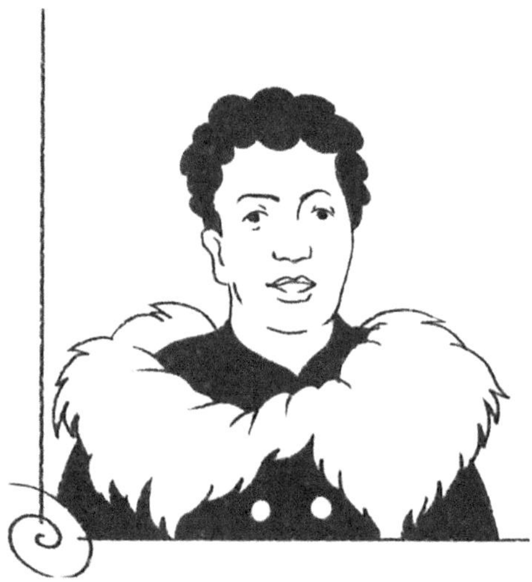

In 1951, a young Black woman was dying of uterine cancer at Johns Hopkins Hospital in the United States. Though there was nothing particularly remarkable about Henrietta Lacks' life, her fatal illness proved to be a major step toward scientific immortality. During surgery, a piece of Henrietta's tumor tissue was taken for testing. At the time, researcher Dr. George Guy worked at this hospital (major hospitals in the United States are traditionally not simply places to heal, but are also medical research centers). Dr. Guy was passionate about the idea of cultivating cells in an artificial laboratory medium (outside the body). However, either due to the lack of nutrient medium, or perhaps some other reason, all of these cells (including cancer cells) would die off within just a few days. Dr. Guy did not give up — he added more and more new ingredients to the medium, including umbilical cord blood and calf germ puree (this sounds like a recipe for a medieval witchcraft potion, does it not?) and even invented a special machine for spinning test tubes in which tissues are cultured (improved analogues are still used in laboratories today). The movement of the liquid medium in the spinning test tubes was supposed to imitate the natural flow of nutrient fluids in a living organism. However, even this ingenious invention was unable to significantly extend the life of the cells. Henrietta Lacks' sample was one of hundreds of those that George Guy attempted to culture using his own system, but it was the first time after many years that he expected to see any success.

Henrietta's cells did not die off after a few days, or even a month, as had been the case with all of Guy's previous samples. Instead, they divided, doubling their number every twenty-four hours. The culture, which was named by an abbreviation of the patient's first and last names, was HeLa, and it was the first truly immortal culture of human cells. Today, the total amount of cells in various biological and medical laboratories around the world numbers in the tens of tons. Although the art of tissue culture has advanced significantly, and researchers have been able to obtain many high-quality cell lines, HeLa continues to be a favorite. This was the emergence of standard (genetically homogenous) cell lines that made modern molecular biology a truly precise science. Before that, any one biological sample was only approximately similar to another, and in the case of a discrepancy in the results of two laboratories working with, for example, human liver cells, scientists could only guess whether it was due to a mistake by one of the research groups or if the two patients' cells really did have different properties due to their different genetic origins.

Immortal cell cultures made biological experiments both repeatable and reproducible. At least, that is what was thought to be the case until very recently. In recent years, research has shown that cancer lines continue to evolve and are acquiring new mutations, even *in vitro*. That is why, after years of separation and cultivation in different laboratories, they can no longer be considered entirely identical to one another. However, in any case, this is the best thing we have so far.

The HeLa culture played a role in the development of many vaccines, including the American vaccine against polio, which put a stop to the spread of this horrific disease in the Western Hemisphere (the Soviet one was obtained through different methods). HeLa has made, and continues to make, priceless contributions to cancer research and the search for new cancer drugs. Of course, the other side of the coin is that this cell line does have some shortcomings. HeLa cells are so stable and undemanding that they easily displace any other cells (including cancer cells) when grown in an artificial medium. The first scandal related to this was during the 1970s, when it suddenly turned out that HeLa cells were present in many cell lines of the American Type Culture Collection, which had been originally grown from the cells of different patients. Although since then many measures have been taken in order to prevent similar mass "infections," to date, the problem has not been entirely resolved.

Henrietta herself died unaware of the truly breakthrough role her cells would play in global science, though the first scientific results using HeLa were obtained during her lifetime. At the time, there were no standards for informed patient consent when it came to using cell or tissue samples. This was compounded by the fact that Henrietta was not a wealthy white woman from high society, but a poor Black woman born into poverty and with little education. No one thought to bother informing her of her cells' extraordinary success. Though pharmaceutical companies made millions, if not billions, of dollars from HeLa, neither Henrietta nor her descendants (she left behind several children) have ever seen a cent of that money. In the end, as with many human stories, it is hard to say whether the ending to this story is happy or sad...

LIFE IN DEVELOPMENT

We began our study of life with the building blocks — the structure of the genome and cell division. But the human body does not simply grow methodically as it increases in size. From conception to maturity, our bodies take a long, winding path of development as we form such wondrous, complex structures as our hands and feet, the ability to perform precise manipulations, a face with muscles that allow us to express thousands of shades of emotion, and, finally, a brain in charge of all of this wealth. This development (known as ontogenesis) is not a purely human privilege. It is a feature of every multicellular organism, to varying degrees. In our culture, we often think of the image of a tiny seed that grows into a new plant. This idea focuses on progress, or development. However, bringing that idea of development in alignment with the idea of the inheritance of genetic traits has not been such an easy task in biology.

Even non-scientists are able to understand genetics on the level of "one organism = one genotype." People of all walks of life talk about genes for eye or hair color, and every new parent has heard the question "Who does the baby look like?" plenty of times. But once we bring up the idea of development, there are suddenly a lot of questions.

A zygote is the very first cell of your body formed by a sperm cell and an egg fusing together. The person you become twenty years later shares the very same genome, but it is hard to imagine two organisms with less in common! The skin cells of one person can look like the skin cells of another, even if they have different genotypes, but those skin cells will look nothing like the same person's neurons. Then we come to the rather childish question — what, exactly, do eye color genes have to do with the liver, which does not have eyes at all?

Classical genetics was incapable of answering these questions. But scientists had begun to think of them long before reaching the molecular frontier. During the 1940s, British biologist Conrad Waddington suggested the metaphor of an "epigenetic landscape" to describe the creation of such diverse cell types in the same organism.

Imagine a ball at the top of a mountain. At first, it might end up at any point at the bottom, but as it rolls its way down the slope, the number of potential trajectories will gradually shrink, and at the end there is only one "highly specialized" path with only one possible outcome. That metaphor is a good explanation of the sequential specialization of tissues during embryonic development, but says nothing about the mechanisms behind that effect. It was not until the end of the twentieth century that biologists were able to explain them (and not in full).

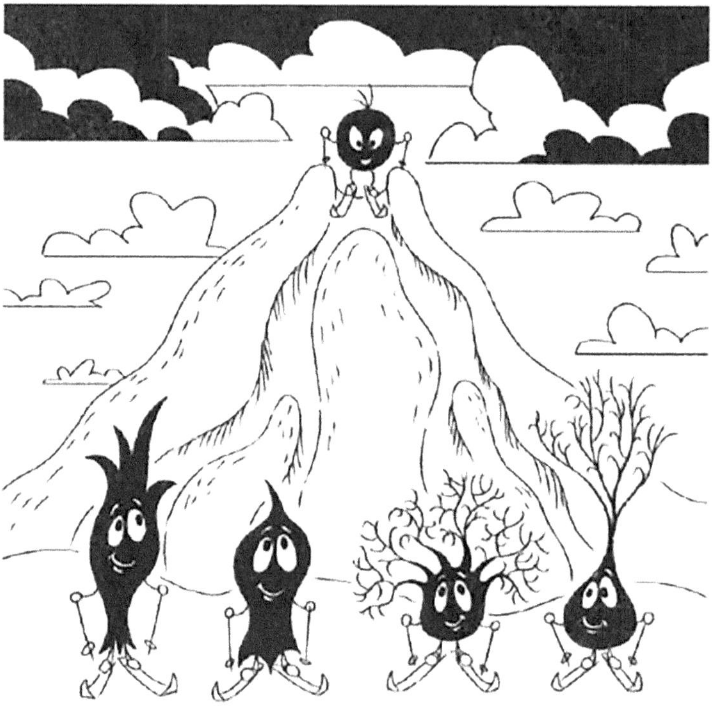

Figure 13. The epigenetic landscape. The descendants of the same cell, a zygote formed by the fusion of a sperm cell and an egg cell, create all of the cells in our body – from neurons to white blood cells. They share the same genome but have different epigenomes, which explains the differences between them.

It turns out that genes within the genome contain special molecular markers, similar to a hashtag used on social media. In simple terms, genes with a #liver marker will be active in the liver, while genes with the #neuron marker will be active in the brain. Do you recall that in the chapter on the genome we talked about how different parts of the genome are packed at different densities? The epigenetic markers (hello, Waddington!) determine whether a gene in a certain cell type will be densely packed and hidden, or instead active and available for binding with transcription regulation proteins. Some of these epigenetic markers are related to chemical changes to the DNA (methylation of cytosine residues in a gene lead to it "turning off"). Other modifications will affect histone proteins. The attachment of acetic acid residue (acetylation) to a histone reduces its positive charge and weakens the interaction between the protein and the DNA. As a result, the gene becomes more accessible for interaction with transcription factors, and its activity increases.

Now, to answer that "childish question" from earlier — what do eye color genes have to do with liver cells? Nothing at all. Those genes are inactive in the liver cells.

Unlike the stable genotype, epigenotypes are constantly changing. They change from one type to another within the cell, ensuring their specialization, and they also change over the course of human body development.

Mutations in the cancer cell genome disrupt its marker system — the epigenome. Heightened (hyper)methylation of oncosuppressor genes and decreased methylation of oncogenes leads to changes in their activity in the tumor, even in the absence of mutations, changing many properties in the transformed cell. In many ways, cancer is more similar to embryonic, germinal tissues than to the mature and specialized cells that produced it. As we discussed earlier, many tumors even express embryonic proteins, which are usually "closed off" for expression in an adult body. However, "similar" does not mean "the same." If tumors were to reproduce at the same rate as embryonic tissue, they would lose their main feature — the ability to develop and consequently become more complex.

A carcinoma will not grow another arm or a third eye. From the very beginning, right up to the end, the tumor will continue to be a chaotic conglomerate of cells. That heterogeneity and specialization, which still exists in the tumor, is only a pathological shadow of normal tissue differentiation in a healthy organ. A malignant neoplasm aims to achieve eternal self-production, but the price of that "immortality" is the inability to develop.

This is why it is impossible for humans to directly borrow tumor cells' molecular strategies. Hardly anyone would be interested in eternal "existence" as cellular broth, devoid of any feelings, consciousness, or movement. Extending the life of the human body involves preserving all of its complexities, which are notably absent in tumor tissues.

Though cancer epigenetics is still a very young science, some of its discoveries already look very promising for clinical use. Sometimes, a primary tumor goes undetected, until the patient goes to the doctor with secondary tumors from metastases in different parts of the body. In order to choose an effective cancer treatment, it is crucial to know the exact tissue origin of the cancer (in order to determine sensitivity to hormonal therapy, among other reasons). Routine cytological analysis cannot always answer this question, because in the course of returning to a near-embryonic state, many cancer cells will take on individual features which are inherent to the tissues that produced them. However, the genome's epigenetic markers are more conservative. Of course, cancer regeneration will lead to changes in the epigenome as well but, fortunately, only some of the genes will be affected, while the others will retain markers in the locations of the original, healthy tissue. Thus, by comparing the location of these markers in the tumor genome with the "epigenetic profiles" of already known healthy tissue, it is possible to accurately predict the origin and location of the primary tumor and select an appropriate treatment.

Changes to the epigenetic markers are associated with the corresponding proteins' pathological activity, for example, DNA methyltransferase enzymes, which tag certain DNA fragments with methyl groups. Clinical trials are currently underway studying the effectiveness of using inhibitors on these proteins to prevent malignant cell rearrangement.

FACT: A tumor is incapable of developing and forming complex structures. Human immortality or longevity requires the regular renewal of complex structures (tissues and organs).

STEM CELLS – THE SOURCE OF ETERNAL YOUTH AND CANCER ALIKE

It is possible to observe the typical fifty to seventy cellular divisions in mature cells in a laboratory setting, and this is not an experiment that takes a lot of time, but the human lifespan is much longer than that. How can we reconcile these two facts? "Mature" is the key word in this riddle. During the early twentieth century, a brilliant Russian (and later American) histologist named Alexander Maksimov demonstrated that in the adult organisms of humans and animals, some mature (non-cancerous!) cells retain features of embryonic cells. Later on, it turned out that these cells continue synthesizing telomerase, and when necessary are capable of lengthening the ends of their chromosomes. These cells became known as "stem cells." By dividing stem cells, the adult organism is able to replace old cells that have died of apoptosis with new, "young" cells. As a rule, one of the daughter cells formed by such a progenitor cell through cellular division will remain a stem cell, while the second will take the path of specialization differentiation, so that the main population of stem cells is not consumed as the organism renews itself.

Unfortunately, the quantity and quality of stem cells will decrease with age, for reasons that are not always clear to scientists. Most likely, this is one of the reasons for the body's overall aging, and gradually slower recovery process. If we could learn how to maintain the body's stem cell population at youthful levels, it would probably allow us to prolong the human lifespan while making it much more productive and healthier. We need to learn the lessons of immortality not from cancerous tumors, but from our own bodies.

According to some data, stem cells are also capable of renewing nerve tissue, meaning that if we were able to "harness" them successfully, we would be capable of preserving both physical and intellectual abilities, which in many people tend to deteriorate with age. Stem cells are also used in cancer treatment. In addition to "solid" tumors, which are the main focus of this book, there are also "fluid" cancers of the organs that form blood, commonly referred to as "blood cancers" or leukemia. For many leukemias, the only treatment available has long been the complete destruction of the patient's own hematopoietic system (bone marrow) and a bone marrow transplant from a donor. But this is a very complicated, costly operation, the success of which largely depends on the degree of genetic match between the donor and patient. In recent decades, an alternative has developed. In some cases, rather than transplanting another person's bone marrow, doctors are able to "graft" hematopoietic stem cells, which can recreate normal hematopoietic tissue.

The search for a way to extend human life is moving in various directions, and it is still hard to say exactly what idea will pan out, but the approach of using our own body's natural abilities to renew itself (by renewing the stem cell population) looks the most promising today.

The main obstacle on the path toward widespread use of cellular technology in medicine remains the difficulty of obtaining human stem cells. For the past few decades, researchers have been attempting to learn how to reprogram mature human cells back into stem cells. After all, they share the same genome, while the epigenome, as we learned earlier, is something it takes on later. A few years ago, researchers were able to turn back time when they managed to find the conditions (a set of transcription factors) to be activated in order to reprogram mature cells into stem cells. In 2008, *Science* magazine recognized the creation of these induced stem cells as one of the most important discoveries of the year, and in 2012 the same discovery was awarded the Nobel Prize, shared by Briton John Gurdon and Shinya Yamanaka of Japan. In the history of the Nobel Prize, it is rare for such a short time period to go by between the discovery and the award. Today, research groups around the world are working on developing a more effective and safer way to turn mature cells into stem cells, but that laboratory method still has a long way to go before being considered a full-fledged biotechnology. The main problem is that stem cells reprogrammed *in vitro* are still too carcinogenic to be recommended for clinical applications. However, we assume that this is a surmountable challenge. What is much worse is the fact that it seems that "natural" stem cells also have a significant potential to form malignant tumors. After all, it is stem cells in the brain that lead to glioblastomas and other tumors of the nervous system, while embryonic stem cells that go astray within the adult body can cause teratocarcinomas. We have yet to understand how the body manages these "eternally young" cells and prevents them from turning into cancer. As is the case with division, here we can see that the human body's natural process of growth and renewal is inextricably linked to the risk of malignant transformation, just as on the psychological and moral level, free will can drive a person to either good or evil.

All of the above applies to normal stem cells in a healthy body. However, research in the last few decades suggests that cancerous tumors may have their own stem cells, with higher potential for malignancy and greater ability to divide than other tumor cells. Scientists working in this area believe that cancer that recurs after what appeared to be successful treatment may be related to the fact that the drugs were more effective against "normal" cancer cells, but not effective enough against stem cells. Remember, all it takes is literally a pair of surviving cells to create a new tumor. Today, researchers are actively testing this hypothesis and trying to develop new approaches to cancer treatment specifically focused on destroying malignant stem cells.

SUMMARY

In this chapter, we learned that the cause of malignant tumor growth is not only the acceleration of the cell cycle, but also disruption of the regulation of programmed cell death — apoptosis — which allows cells with significant genomic abnormalities to continue dividing, rather than dying off. One of the most common causes of apoptosis disruption in cancer is the mutation of the p53 protein. Another mechanism that supports the “eternal life” of cancerous cell lines is the constant renewal of the ends of the chromosomes, or telomeres. A special enzyme called telomerase, which is normally only active in embryonic tissue and stem cells, is responsible for this renewal. Malignant tumors generally share many features with fetal tissues, and in addition to telomerases, they activate the synthesis of several germline oncofetal proteins, which doctors use to diagnose the disease based on their tumor marker proteins. However, there is one critical difference between embryonic tissue and malignant tumors. The “immortality” of cancer tissues is achieved at the expense of being able to specialize, which means that the tissue cannot develop, whereas the key to human immortality is probably technology that harnesses the body’s own natural capacity for self-renewal, for example, stem cells. Now is a good time to ask ourselves about the “cost” of cancer cells’ malignant transformations, as accelerating division and growth is a very energy-intensive process. In the next chapter, we will look at the features of malignant tumors’ biochemical metabolism and the outlook for cancer treatment with diets and supplements.

Chapter 5
QUESTIONS ABOUT METABOLISM AND MYTHS ABOUT "EATING WELL"

Eating a balanced diet is the easiest and most obvious way that the average person can influence their body. Not everyone will be brave enough to cut, stitch, or even inject something into their bodies, but it is extremely easy to eat something "healthy" or avoid eating something "unhealthy." It comes as no surprise that many of the more optimistic myths about cancer that promise a quick and full recovery revolve around the idea of a proper or "therapeutic" diet.

In this chapter, we will examine myths about cancer as a disease primarily affecting people with a sweet tooth and discuss the intricacies of the acid–alkaline balance that supporters of a baking soda–based cancer treatment are trying to achieve. In order to separate reasonable ideas about diets that help prevent the development of some types of cancer from fantastical ideas about nutrition as a panacea, we will have to discuss metabolism, that is, the dynamic exchange of substances and energy in living systems.

We will also take a (culinary) look at some interesting habits around the world. Russia seems to have mostly avoided this trend, but for some time in the United States, there was once a widespread idea that sharks do not get cancer, so shark cartilage is capable of curing the disease. Where did this myth come from? Are there really animals out there that do not get cancer, and if so, should we eat them?

THE SWEET FUEL OF LIFE

Some time ago, there was a popular joke on the Internet that is useful to keep in mind when we study cause and effect in complex systems: "I am the most important — I know everyone!" said Facebook. "No, I am the most important. I know everything about everyone!" said Google. "No, I am the most important — I am everything!" said the Internet. "Well, well, well..." said electricity, as it blinked...

When we think about gene copying and protein synthesis, we cannot lose sight of the fact that these fascinating macromolecular games of life require "material support" as a constant flow of matter and energy. Without electricity, there is no Internet, and without metabolism, there is no life.

Exchanging matter and energy in a living organism is something like an exchange at the market. Any change — growth, movement, reproduction — requires resources and raises the question: who is paying for this? In each cell, there are hundreds if not thousands of reactions, just like at the market, where people exchange goods and services. History shows us that the effectiveness of market exchanges will increase dramatically if there is an exchange equivalent — money. Surprisingly, billions of years before human society even existed, the biomechanics of evolution followed the exact same path, and most biochemical reactions used molecules of adenosine triphosphate (ATP) as "universal energy currency." Historically, paper money was tied to the value of precious metals — the gold standard — but in recent years many economists have begun to discuss the idea that a single global currency, should one ever exist, should be tied to the value of energy — in which case, the analogy between money and ATP would come full circle. In essence, this molecule is nothing more than a rechargeable chemical battery, a kind of molecular charger.

ATP molecules are formed when their predecessor, the adenosine diphosphate (ADP) molecule, adds a third phosphate residue and stores energy as a high-energy bond. If the energy reserve must be used, the reaction will go in the other direction. The ATP molecule will disintegrate into ADP and a phosphoric acid residue, thus "discharging" and using the energy released during the destruction of the chemical bond for a variety of the body's needs, from synthesizing new molecules to ensuring the movement of sperm's flagella (tails). Most biochemical reactions in the body are accompanied by either ATP synthesis and energy storage, or ATP decomposition and energy use.

If we were to draw a map of all of the biochemical reactions in the human cells that we know of today, it would look like an enormous network with hundreds if not thousands of nodes. It would be easy to get lost in this labyrinth, even for an expert, but in the context of cancer, we will only be looking at one: the most ancient and conservative part of the network, that is, the glucose oxidation pathway.

The six-carbon sugar glucose is the main product of photosynthesis in both bacteria and plants, and is capable of using or "storing" sunlight energy in the form of organic compounds. It is also the main nutrient for all living things, including humans. Oxidation or "burning" of glucose in the cells is the main source of energy for "recharging" ATP molecules. In terms of energy exchange, a living cell is like a thermal power plant that transfers energy stored as chemical bonds in the organic gas and oil molecules into a more accessible and effective form of electrical energy.

Life appeared on our planet when its atmosphere was almost devoid of oxygen, and for many millions of years, it existed in such anaerobic conditions, until the oldest photosynthesizing organisms — blue-green algae — began to radically change the molecular composition of the air. That took place about 2.5 billion years ago, and is known as the "Great Oxidation Event" in scientific literature.

One souvenir of that ancient, oxygen-free time is the fact that we have two metabolic pathways for glucose oxidation: ancient, oxygen-free glycolysis and more modern, oxidative phosphorylation.

Both exist in the cell, complementing and at times "substituting" one another.

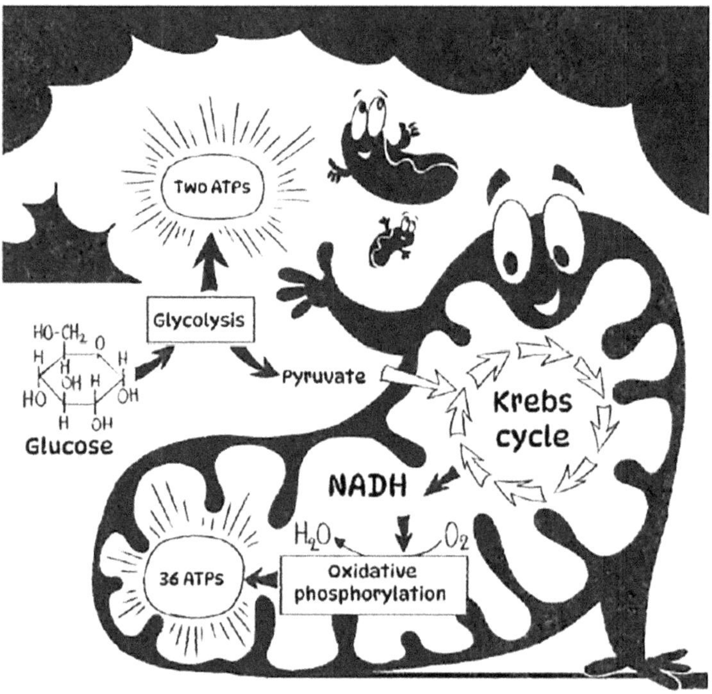

Figure 14. Mitochondria are like tiny power plants inside our cells. They "burn" glucose into carbon dioxide and water (just as thermal power plants burn natural gas or coal), and store released energy as ATP molecules. Metabolic abnormalities in cancer cells are yet another key sign of cancer (see Figure 1).

During oxygen-free glycolysis, only two ATP molecules are synthesized using one glucose molecule to create lactic acid, or lactate. On the other hand, full oxidation with oxygen, during which the glucose molecule creates carbon dioxide and water, produces thirty-eight

ATP molecules, which is significantly more than in oxygen-free glycolysis. Since this pathway was so advantageous to organisms that use oxygen, it comes as no surprise that they have nearly entirely displaced ancient oxygen-free bacteria, relegating them to the very margins of modern ecosystems.

Glycolysis takes place right in the cell's cytoplasm, while oxidative phosphorylation reactions take place within special organelles, the mitochondria.

It was this feature of glucose metabolism in cancer cells that led to the "baking soda" myth and the idea that we can cure cancer by giving up sweets.

FACT: In addition to ATP, human cells use other molecules to store energy (also known as macroenergetic molecules). For example, guanosine triphosphate molecules play a very important role in regulating the functions of many proteins.

HOW THE WARBURG EFFECT ALLOWS US TO SEE THE TUMOR

During the nineteenth century, while observing yeast, French researcher Louis Pasteur described a phenomenon that would later be known as the "Pasteur effect": when yeast is intensively aerated, the fermentation process (oxygen-free glycolysis) in the broth stops, but the yeast begins to grow much faster. It was revealed that one single organism (the yeast) can metabolize in different ways, depending on conditions (oxygen deficiency or excess). Later, the same observation — the type of metabolism depending on access to oxygen — was observed in human cells, though unlike yeast they of course cannot survive in a completely oxygen-free environment.

One example of the Pasteur effect that many of us have encountered when we begin exercising is the burning sensation in our muscles during strength training. That feeling is caused by the accumulation of lactic acid, or lactate, which is the main product of oxygen-free metabolism. A weekend warrior's circulatory system simply cannot cope with the increased burden, and the blood does not have time to deliver enough oxygen to the muscles and remove the byproducts of metabolism, which is why our muscles switch to glycolytic metabolism and "acidify" with lactate. Lactic acid irritates our muscle-tissue receptors, which we feel as a burning sensation. If we begin to train regularly, our muscles will grow new blood vessels, our heart will begin to contract harder, and our muscle tissues will return to normal respiration — with oxygen. This is how most healthy tissues behave.

During the twentieth century, when German scientist Otto Warburg began studying the metabolic features of cancer cells, he noticed that oxygen-free metabolism (glycolysis) predominated, regardless of how intensively the tumor was supplied with oxygen. This phenomenon was named the "Warburg effect." Warburg was so impressed by the regularity he observed in a wide variety of tumors, that he suggested that a metabolic disorder was at the root of malignant transformation.

The first half of the twentieth century was the "golden age" of biochemistry. Thus, scientists were enthusiastic about a universal biochemical explanation for how cancer develops. However, after the discovery of DNA and the role of mutations in malignant transformations, that hypothesis (which was very sound and fully in line with the scientific developments of its time) was ruled out by biological science, though this did not prevent it from remaining widespread in alternative medicine circles.

Despite the fact that with the advent of molecular biology, classical biochemistry was temporarily relegated to the back burner in cancer research, Warburg's discovery did not go unnoticed, and became the foundation for one of the most sensitive methods of clinical diagnosis of malignant tumors — positron emission tomography (PET).

Before the advent of PET, a doctor who had removed a primary tumor and prescribed chemotherapy could only guess whether all of the disease foci had been destroyed, or whether there were still invisible and undetectable microtumors of metastases that could start to grow again at any time. All the doctor and patient could do was wait and hope for the best. Today, PET allows us to see all tumors present in the body, and, if for any reason some of them are inoperable, we can monitor them "in real time" to see what kind of effects chemotherapy or radiation is having on them. We can see if the tumor is shrinking or continuing to grow at the same rate, and whether new metastases have appeared or not.

Essentially, in a PET scan, a patient is given a solution of radioactively labeled glucose analog (the dose of radiation is not dangerous), waits a bit for the molecules to distribute evenly throughout the body, and then is placed on a scanner that registers radiation from various parts of the body. Healthy cells will absorb glucose with more or less the same intensity, displaying the body's "background radiation." But if there is a tumor present, greedily absorbing glucose, it will show up on the scan as a dark spot. (The metaphorical "greed" here is in fact quite material on a molecular level — the tumor cells will actively produce a protein, glucose transporter GLUT1.) This is an excellent method for detecting microtumors and metastases that cannot be detected by other means, and is used for both diagnosis and treatment quality control.

Unfortunately, PET also has its own limitations. Inflamed tissue often behaves similarly (we will discuss why later on), capturing more glucose than healthy tissues. If there are any doubts as to whether changes in signal intensity are due to a malignant transformation or inflammation, the patient is usually given a course of antibiotics and the scan is repeated.

Practical applications of the Warburg effect opened a new chapter in laboratory diagnostics, but the question still remains: why do tumor cells prefer the more ancient metabolic pathway of glycolysis to the more efficient oxidation?

The hypothesis generally accepted today is that while cells "lose" in reactions aimed at extracting energy, they make gains in synthetic pathways during glycolysis. Intermediary products are used to produce amino acids and nucleotides, the building blocks of proteins and nucleic acids, respectively, whose synthesis is no less important for a rapidly growing and frequently dividing cell than ATP production. This hypothesis is supported by the fact that an effect similar to the Warburg effect is observed in normal but very rapidly dividing embryonic tissues. Thus, rearranging the metabolism does not lead to changes in cellular behavior, as Warburg initially suggested, but, on the contrary, frequently dividing cells choose the metabolic pathway that can supply them with both energy and building materials for growth.

In addition to this basic explanation, tumors have many other reasons to use glycolysis. For example, it has been demonstrated that an acidic environment created in the tumor due to the heightened lactate content promotes the spread of metastases. Lactic acid depresses anti-cancer activity in innate immune cells known as macrophages, while cancer cells' insatiability means that they actively absorb glucose from their environment, leaving the main acquired immunity cells — T-cells, also called T-lymphocytes—"hungry," which also weakens the local immune response.

FACT: Genome abnormalities leading to accelerated cancer cell division and the disruption of cell death mechanisms go hand in hand with a general metabolic restructuring within the tumor.

SYMBIOSIS — THE ART OF SURVIVING TOGETHER

Otto Warburg had to work with rather large tumor tissue samples — biochemical methods were not particularly precise during his time. Today, scientists are able to break a tumor down into individual cells and study their properties, literally one at a time. By applying modern methods for studying metabolic pathways to tumors, they discovered that on the microlevel this metabolism has nuances that Warburg simply did not have the opportunity to analyze.

In recent years, we increasingly see expressions in literature on cancer cell biology that we would expect to find in descriptions of the interaction between organisms and the biosphere—"ecosystem," "symbiosis," etc. It turns out that looking at the problem from another perspective — in this case, ecology — we notice many interesting regularities in tumor cell behavior.

We saw earlier that unlike healthy cells, which are subject to a general set of rules within the entire organism, cancer cells are "individualists" and, in a way, each of them could be considered as a separate living being competing with others. However, despite the "individualism" inherent in each cell, they do have a "shared interest"— survival within the organism, which means that they both compete and cooperate among themselves. This leads to a situation similar to that in an animal population, where males compete over females while also cooperating against a common enemy. Unsurprisingly, the survival strategies in a tumor are similar to those of a pack of wolves or a pride of lions.

One example of this strategy is the metabolic specialization of cells, depending on their position within the tumor. Generally, there is a deficit of oxygen (hypoxia) within the tumor, and the cells there process glucose primarily via glycolysis (the Warburg effect). However, it also turns out that the lactate they secrete does not go to waste. It is used by surface cancer cells, which are more effectively supplied with oxygen. They oxidize lactate into carbon dioxide and water, and thus glucose is used much more efficiently by the system than would normally be expected. The tumor surface cells, which are supplied with oxygen, appear to be "disinterested," which looks quite a bit like "real" symbiosis between organisms within this system.

These cells can consume both glucose and lactate with equal efficiency, but they "pass" glucose to the oxygen-deficient cells in the center of the tumor, while contenting themselves with only the lactate produced by the cells on the inside. This behavior is similar to the symbiosis of algae living in the world's oceans at different depths and specializing in absorbing waves of light at a certain frequency, so that the system as a whole is able to use a valuable resource such as sunlight as efficiently as possible.

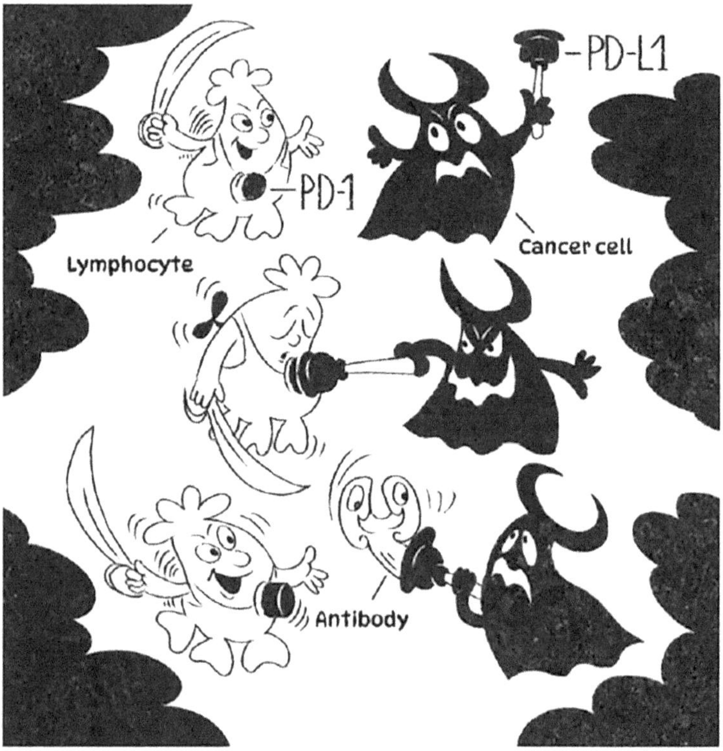

Figure 15. The symbiosis of cancer cells. Cells on the tumor's surface share glucose with those on the inside, and in turn use lactate produced by cells on the inside. This specialization allows cancer to cope with the lack of oxygen, which worsens, as vascular growth (one of the key signs of malignant rearrangement, see Figure 1) does not keep up with tumor growth.

Disrupting the metabolic symbiosis of cancer cells in a tumor might be the foundation for a new type of anti-cancer therapy. What happens if the protein responsible for transporting lactate is blocked, and the inner cells are prevented from secreting it into their environment? It turns out that, in this situation, the surface cells quickly shift and become more "selfish" as they consume resources, and they begin to greedily absorb glucose without allowing it to be passed on. As a result, the cancer cells within the tumor begin to die off due to a lack of nutrients. Scientists are currently studying this approach to cancer treatment.

This is just one of many examples of "metabolic cancer therapy," based on the difference between metabolic processes in healthy and malignant cells. Many pharmacological laboratories are working on such therapies right now. Sometimes, oncologists get a hand from somewhere completely unexpected. As we know, the most common disease related to glucose metabolism disorders is diabetes mellitus. Millions of diabetes patients around the world have been treated for many years, and a wide variety of medical statistics have been collected on them. Recently, it was discovered that the drug metformin, which is prescribed to people with diabetes to control blood sugar levels, has a pronounced anti-cancer effect! Patients taking metformin developed cancerous tumors at much lower rates than the average population, and those who did develop cancer had much higher survival rates. Researchers are now actively testing the potential of this drug for cancer prevention and treatment, and it may soon be recommended for various risk groups.

Of course, scientists do not expect metabolic drugs to be as powerful as traditional chemotherapy, which, in some cases, is enough to beat cancer on its own, but these drugs could be potent adjuvant drugs that strengthen and reinforce other therapies.

FACT: Malignant cells' interaction with both the healthy cells surrounding them and other tumor cells is very significant to cancerous tumors.

HOMEOSTASIS – WHY SIMPLE SOLUTIONS JUST DO NOT WORK

In both the "baking soda" and "sugar" myths about cancer, popular fiction is intricately intertwined with some scientific truths. The Warburg effect causes cancer cells to absorb glucose much more actively than healthy tissue does, and by intensively producing lactic acid, tumors acidify their surrounding environment. This is a fact that scientists and the myth makers can agree on. But the conclusions they reach based on these facts could not be more different. By claiming that it is easy to "acidify" or, on the contrary, "alkalize" the body and kill cancer, by reducing one's intake of glucose with food, the peddlers of "alternative" medicine are focusing their attention on the tumor, losing sight of the fact that it is not growing in a test tube, but in a living human body. A living body differs from a non-living environment not least due to its ability to maintain a constant internal environment, despite interaction with the outside world, and, in particular, despite the ill-conceived treatments provided by "alternative medicine" providers.

Stone or water always takes on the ambient temperature, but mammals are capable of maintaining their body temperature at the same level in both heat and cold. Water will evaporate from a wet dishrag left in the sun within a few minutes, and animals (especially those that have adapted to hot climates) are able to go for days at a time without any water. If we rinse salted pasta several times in clean water, most of the salt will rinse away, but we can safely swim in a river or take a bath, and the salt content of our body will remain the same. The property of living matter to "remain itself" in any conditions is known as homeostasis. This has developed to different degrees in different organisms, but it is in one way or another present in all of us – from bacteria to human beings. Homeostasis is the property that makes it possible for us to have clinical diagnoses. In most healthy people, cardiac muscle activity and blood composition fall within a "normal range," and when the values of some vital signs go beyond this range, it is usually indicative of disease.

Is this an accident? Of course not. In multicellular organisms, life requires the coordination of millions of molecular reactions and biochemical transformations, and in such a complex system, the most important parameters, such as temperature or pH levels, must remain constant in order to avoid complete chaos.

Temperature has a direct influence on the rate of chemical reactions. We all know from high school chemistry class that a temperature increase of 10 °C will lead to a chemical reaction speed that is two to four times faster (the Van 't Hoff rule), but even more importantly for biological systems, a temperature increase of over 40 °C will disrupt normal protein functioning. And since "life is the existence of protein bodies," it ceases when those proteins are destroyed.

But proteins are also sensitive to environmental acidity. Even a slight (by chemical standards) change to this parameter can have a major effect on protein enzyme activity. This is why most human body fluids (blood, lymph, tissue fluid) are buffer solutions. They are capable of neutralizing significant amounts of acid or alkali and maintain a normal pH level (for blood, a slightly alkaline pH of 7.36 to 7.44 is considered normal; the pH of pure distilled water is 7.00).

However, the body's ability to maintain acidity at the same level has little to do with the baking soda myth. Baking soda that we ingest in our food or drinks does not enter the bloodstream and will be neutralized by the acid of gastric juices. In fact, we sometimes feel the process of excess acid being neutralized as heartburn — baking soda was once used to treat digestive disorders until more effective medications were developed. But the acidity of our gastric juices has no effect whatsoever on the basic biochemical parameters of our blood — and that is a good thing! Otherwise, the slightest case of gastritis with either increased or decreased acidity (after all, gastritis is just an extra glass of lemon juice) would kill us all! Drinking large amounts of baking soda solution can upset digestion (digesting proteins require an acidic environment), but blood indicators and the composition of the tissue fluid surrounding the tumor will not change in any way.

Blood sugar levels are more flexible parameters than temperature or acidity, which is why "sugar tests" are usually done on an empty stomach. It is quite normal for blood sugar levels to rise after a meal, though a drop in blood sugar below a certain level can be a sign of distress accompanied by obvious symptoms, such as weakness, dizziness and, in severe cases, a loss of consciousness and coma.

Fortunately, these cases are very rare and usually indicative of a serious illness. In a healthy organism, there is a reliable and "foolproof" defense system which can only be broken into at the risk of death. The human body's main glucose consumer is the "control center"—the brain – and it will be provided with nutrition at literally "any cost." Thus, a person might avoid sweets entirely and eat almost exclusively protein (meat and fish) as we see in some fad diets or people who live near the Arctic Circle, and their blood sugar level will remain the same as anyone else's, as the excess amino acids will simply be converted into glucose. Beyond special diets, even someone who is literally dying of starvation will have a rather high blood sugar level right up until the last moment. The body will consume both fat tissue and muscle tissue, just to provide the brain with enough nutrition to figure a way out of this threatening situation.

It is pointless (and dangerous!) to attempt to influence our health by adjusting such basic parameters of the human body as the pH balance and blood sugar levels. However, if you change your eating habits correctly, you can actually normalize your body's metabolic processes, which will reduce your chances of getting a whole range of cancers.

FACT: The main mechanism for maintaining homeostasis in living systems is the mechanism for negative feedback, the pancreas, which is constantly working to bring the entire system back to its original state in any case of deviation. For example, when blood sugar levels rise, the pancreas begins producing the hormone insulin. Insulin increases the uptake of glucose into the liver cells, fat tissue, and muscles, which causes blood sugar to drop to a normal level. In people with diabetes, this regulatory system is disrupted.

Mitochondria – the story of a single organelle

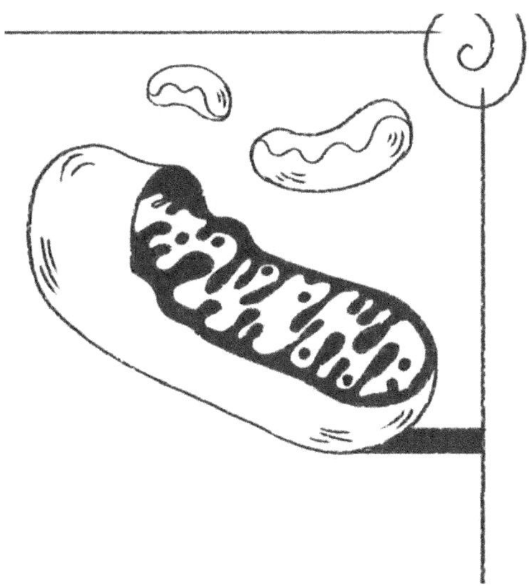

We already discussed mitochondria in the chapter on apoptosis. The destruction of these organelles triggers the activation of the planned-cell-death mechanisms. However, mitochondria's main function in the cell is still energetic in nature. The inner membrane of mitochondria contains a protein complex known as ATP synthase, which uses energy obtained during glucose oxidation to synthesize ATP.

Whenever we speak about multicellular organisms, we must also remember the issue of symbiosis — mutually beneficial cooperation between living things. However, it turns out that the nuclear cell, which is a basic unit of life, is itself an example of symbiosis between several cells, which have partially "dissolved" into one (cell) structure, while retaining some features of isolation. Unlike other organelles, mitochondria and chloroplasts (in plants) are not simply macromolecule complexes, but ancient bacteria which inhabited the cells of nuclear organisms so long ago that even their genomes have partially merged with ours. Despite the fact that mitochondria have their own DNA (circular, as in the case of bacteria), many genes necessary for them to function normally are preserved in the nucleus.

Assumptions on the symbiotic nature of the links between mitochondria and the cells of nuclear organisms (eukaryotes) were already being made in the late nineteenth century, but it was not until the discoveries of the twentieth century that scientists were able to prove such a bold hypothesis. Although many areas of evolutionary biology have traditionally complained about the lack or deficit of intermediary forms, this is one area where mitochondrial theory has been rather lucky. In nature, there are still organisms that mimic the intermediary forms between bacteria and the formation of mitochondria. For example, the primitive amoeba *Pelomyxa* does not have mitochondria, but it does store endosymbiotic bacteria in its cytoplasm, which perform the same energetic functions. Additionally, it turns out that, even in multicellular organisms, mitochondria sometimes migrate from cell to cell, demonstrating their relative independence.

Inheriting mitochondria is different from the way we usually inherit things in sexual reproduction, when half of the new organism's genome comes from the father, and half comes from the mother. When the egg is fertilized, only the sperm's nuclear DNA gets inside the egg, but the father's mitochondria do not. This is why mitochondria are only inherited from the female line, and, amazingly, all of the female lines present in humanity today seem to go back to a single woman who lived in Africa about two hundred thousand years ago. In popular literature, she has been nicknamed "mitochondrial Eve," though the researchers who discovered this phenomenon initially suggested calling her Lucky Mother. This woman was the only one whose female descendants have survived to the present day. But we should not confuse "mitochondrial Eve" with Eve from the Bible. There is no doubt that there were other women who lived at the same time as her, but their mitochondrial DNA simply has not survived this long (perhaps they had only sons and no daughters), though modern people may have inherited other fragments of nuclear DNA from them.

In the small mitochondrial genome, as in the "large" nuclear genome, sometimes there are breakages that lead to the development of severe diseases, such as Barth syndrome, Leigh syndrome, mitochondrial encephalomyopathy, and special myoclonic epilepsy. These genetic disorders are inevitably passed from a woman with defective mitochondria to her children.

Most mitochondrial diseases are untreatable. However, a recent medical technique that has made it possible to prevent them has been approved in the United Kingdom, and the rest of the world is likely to follow suit. In essence, the technique is a type of *in vitro* fertilization in which the nucleus of the mother's egg cell containing a mitochondrial defect is transferred to a healthy donor egg, and then fertilized as usual. A child conceived through this method will in fact have three parents — two "nuclear" and one "mitochondrial" but, more importantly, they will be completely free of developing any maternal pathology! This method is a great leap forward in improving human health and a joy for many people who have taken a responsible approach to parenting and wish to avoid passing on any diseases to their children.

YOU ARE WHAT YOU EAT

There are many old, well-known recommendations for leading a healthy lifestyle — some of which are even rooted in fact — that have taken on new meaning when it comes to cancer prevention. For many people, the goal of "being healthy" is simply too abstract, but it is hard to argue with the goal of "not getting cancer." There are many recommendations for "anti-cancer" nutrition, based on many studies on the relationship between cancer and lifestyle.

Most importantly, doctors recommend not overeating and watching your weight. Increased body mass raises your risk of cardiovascular disease as well as many cancers, such as breast cancer (in post-menopausal women), colon cancer, myeloma, pancreatic cancer, uterine cancer, etc. In developed countries, such as the United Kingdom, doctors have ranked obesity as the second most important cancer risk factor after smoking.

We do not yet fully understand exactly how excess weight affects malignant neoplasms, but we can assume that it is related to regulatory functions in the fat tissue. We often think of fat as a passive substance that serves little purpose other than storing nutrients, but that is not the case. Fat tissue plays a role in metabolizing many biologically active substances — hormones and growth factors that influence cellular division and might promote the formation of malignant tumors. Eating a balanced diet along with moderate physical activity will normalize the body's metabolic and regulatory processes and reduce your risk of developing a tumor.

A diet high in fast carbohydrates often leads to excess weight, and this may be one explanation for the myth that cancer is a disease that primarily affects those with a sweet tooth. However, at a normal weight, eating sugar has no effect on one's probability of developing cancer. The risk factor is not the sugar but being overweight — so if weight is not a problem for you, eating a second piece of cake or candy will not increase your cancer risk. Eat up and enjoy!

When it comes to modern dietary recommendations, the anti-cancer diet involves reducing your consumption of red meat (beef, pork, and lamb) and processed meat products (sausage and bacon) as well as lowering your salt intake.

Red meat's carcinogenic effect is thought to be related to the fact that animal muscle fibers contain a lot of heme iron (the namesake of the blood protein that carries oxygen, hemoglobin). Heme iron is what makes meat from mammals look "red," unlike the white meat of birds and reptiles. Excess heme iron is released from meat during digestion, which damages the surrounding cells and contributes to their malignant transformation, which is why excessive consumption of red meat increases our risk of cancer in the digestive organs — the stomach, intestines, and pancreas. White meat from poultry and fish, which contain much less heme iron, does not have a carcinogenic effect. Nutritionists suggest eating no more than one and a half pounds of red meat per week, or about three servings, and to consume fresh meat rather than processed foods, which contain heme iron as well as high levels of salt. Cooking salt in itself also has a carcinogenic effect. Excessive salt intake has been reliably linked to a heightened risk of stomach cancer.

"Positive" nutrition recommendations include eating more raw fruits and vegetables (at least five servings per day) and enriching your diet with foods high in plant fiber. Eating fruits and vegetables lowers your risk of lung, oral, and laryngeal cancers. Contrary to popular belief, a deficit in natural nutrients cannot be compensated for with artificial supplements. Vitamins from the pharmacy, unlike a diet rich in fruits and vegetables, will not make you less likely to develop cancer. There is, however, one exception to that rule — vitamin D. Regularly taking this vitamin, which tends to be deficient in adults who primarily work indoors, will significantly lower your risk of breast cancer, and, according to a 2014 meta-analysis, it will reduce your risk of death from all cancers by 12 percent.

A diet rich in plant fiber will lower your risk of developing colon cancer. On one hand, the fiber increases the volume of your stool and shortens the time that harmful substances in digested food interact with your intestinal walls. On the other hand, it promotes the reproduction of beneficial intestinal bacteria. However, based on various studies over the past decade, the latter is so important to our health that it deserves its own chapter. The effect of other foods, like green tea, dairy products, and soy products on cancer risk is still up in the air.

FACT: For years, doctors have suspected that artificial sugar substitutes, such as saccharin and aspartame, may be carcinogenic, though epidemiological studies have not confirmed that fear. Consuming these products is no longer seen as a cancer risk.

GERMS ARE RIGHT AT HOME

It is interesting to see how language reacts to changing scientific concepts. Previously, we referred to the microorganisms living in the digestive tract as "microflora," a term which has now been replaced by "microbiome." "Microflora" gives the connotation of something simple, optional, decorative, almost like flowers on the windowsill. "Microbiome" is a broad term that alludes to the existence of an entire parallel ecosystem within our own organism that is living and developing according to its own rules, but which also has a significant influence on our lives and health. According to microbiologists, there are as many microorganisms (bacteria, viruses, fungi) in the human body as there are cells. Without the microbiome, the human body cannot function properly.

When we are born, our gut is sterile, and we receive our first microbes for our microbiome from our mother's milk. By the age of about three years, a child has developed a full ecosystem of microorganisms. This is one of the reasons why intestinal infections are so dangerous in early childhood. As adults, the bacteria of our microbiome coordinate and resist any outside "invasions," but in infants this line of defense is only beginning to form. Prolonged breastfeeding is a major factor in forming a healthy microbiome in children during their first year of life. The digestible oligosaccharides in human milk, which support the growth of good bacteria, such as *Bifidobacterium longum infantis*, make up about 8 percent of a woman's milk. The profile of these oligosaccharides is unique for each woman, which, in turn, determines the individuality of the infant microbiome.

The microbiome has a major effect on the formation of a child's immune system, which is why it is harmful to take antibiotics unless absolutely necessary, as they can kill both pathogens and beneficial microorganisms. That can lead to long-term negative consequences, including the development of asthma and eczema. Bacteria in a healthy microbiome play a crucial role in normal digestion — they inactivate enzymes, hormones, and toxins present in food, break down bile acids, neutralize allergens, and promote the absorption of vitamins D and B12, calcium, and iron in the gut, while synthesizing vitamins B1, B2, B6, B12, C, K, and H, and nicotinic, pantothenic, and folic acids. However, not all bacteria capable of multiplying in the digestive tract are always beneficial to humans.

Many people have *Helicobacter pylori* living in their gut. For most carriers, this does not cause any problems, but in some people it causes ulcers, which in turn can increase their risk of stomach cancer. According to various estimates, 65 to 80 percent of all gastric cancers are related to this infection, though the disease only occurs in two out of every one hundred carriers. Once again, this confirms that concomitant factors (for example, smoking and eating habits) play an important role in the development of the disease. Stomach cancer is insidious, and in the early stages, when it is very treatable, symptoms do not differ from those of a mild exacerbation of gastritis or ulcer, and people who frequently suffer from these problems are unlikely to pay much attention to it. Patients who suffer from chronic gastrointestinal diseases should have a regular check-up with specialists and undergo gastroscopy in order to ensure that any cancer is diagnosed early on.

The discovery that gastritis and stomach ulcers are infectious diseases impressed the scientific community so much that in 2005, Australian scientists Barry Marshall and Robin Warren won the Nobel Prize for it. Nonetheless, the road to recognition was not easy. Initially, the medical community was dismissive of the idea that stomach ulcers were infectious in nature. Experiments on laboratory animals failed, one after another, and in the end, in a moment of desperation, Barry Marshall himself drank a bacterial culture to demonstrate the connection between *Helicobacter pylori* and the disease. Very quickly, he developed typical signs of severe gastritis, which he was then able to cure with a fourteen-day course of antibiotics. The results of this self-sacrificing experiment were published in the *Medical Journal of*

Australia and became one of the journal's most cited articles since its founding.

Very few microbes are capable of surviving in the acidic environment of our gastric juices (this is why doctors were not convinced that gastritis and ulcers could be caused by *Helicobacter pylori* bacteria). The large intestine, however, is a completely different story, and home to a huge number of various types of microorganisms. The predominance of some ensures good digestion and good health, while the excessive presence of others might cause the development of obesity, chronic illness, and cancer.

In recent years, experiments have shown that, contrary to popular belief, changes to the microflora might be a cause, rather than an effect, of obesity. When bacteria from obese mice were added to the intestines of mice without microbiota, the mice began to gain weight faster than when the microbiota from thin mice were transplanted into their intestines. Moreover, it turns out that when scientists know the makeup of a person's microbiota, they are able to predict whether the person is obese or not, with 90 percent accuracy.

Colorectal cancer is often associated with an overgrowth of *fusobacterium*, *Streptococcus gallolyticus*, some members of the Enterobacteriaceae family, and enterotoxigenic strains of *Bacteroides fragilis*. These bacteria secrete substances that irritate the intestinal wall, causing chronic inflammation, while beneficial bacteria, such as *Lactobacillus reuteri*, are able to synthesize anti-inflammatory substances. In people who consume a primarily plant-based diet, the microbiome is dominated by bacteria that break down polysaccharides, notably Bacteroidetes, which can also protect the host from developing local or systemic inflammation.

Whether healthy or pathological, the makeup of the microbiome in our digestive tract determines our risk of developing cancers of the digestive tract, and also the effectiveness of anti-cancer therapy. Laboratory animals that have received antibiotics or were artificially deprived of an intestinal microbiota developed resistance to chemotherapy drugs, such as 5-fluorouracil, irinotecan, oxaliplatin, gemcitabine, and methotrexate.

Both traditional chemotherapy and the newest types of immunotherapies, which we will discuss in the following chapters of this book, show varying efficacy depending on the structure of the microbiome. Researchers have demonstrated that taking antibacterial drugs to treat an infection during cancer treatment will disrupt the gut microflora and worsen the response to immunotherapy, while, conversely, introducing beneficial *Akkermansia muciniphila* bacteria to the diets of laboratory animals restores their ability to respond to immunotherapy. Thus, a healthy and balanced microbiome appears to help prevent cancer and also improve response to cancer treatment.

There are several basic ways to support (and restore) healthy diversity in the gut microbiome. The most widely available is to regularly consume both probiotics and prebiotics.

Probiotics are cultures of beneficial microorganisms, most often bifidobacteria and lactobacilli. Prebiotics are substances (substrates) that stimulate the growth of these bacteria, such as inulin, fructose, and galactose oligosaccharides as well as dietary fiber, as we saw earlier. Prebiotics can come as supplements, but they are already found in a variety of foods that can support the growth of good bacteria — whole grains, chicory, legumes, garlic, onions, and bananas.

In recent years, direct methods for "grafting" the right bacteria into the intestine have been developed — microbiota transplants. This method is still in the experimental phase, though many data sets suggest that it is highly effective for treatment for a wide range of serious digestive pathologies. Given the speed with which research on the properties of the human microbiome is developing, in the next few years, we may see the advent of new, more effective methods for controlling and improving digestive conditions available for widespread use. For now, the best thing we can do is eat a healthy, balanced diet.

FACT: The number of diverse genes present in the normal human gut microbiome is 150 times greater than the number of genes in the human genome.

MAGICAL THINKING AND SHARK CARTILAGE

One curious example of how modern myths about cancer often involve ancient magical beliefs is the story of shark cartilage. In some ancient cultures, people believed that eating a lion's heart would make them as strong and brave as a lion but, conversely, a warrior who accidentally ate a rooster killed in a cockfight would run the risk of being killed in battle himself. One would think that in developed countries these beliefs would have been left in the past long ago, but that is not always the case. Just thirty years ago, William Lane and Linda Comac published a book in the United States entitled *Sharks Don't Get Cancer*, which made full use of that magical thinking, with some science-based arguments sprinkled in here and there. Shark cartilage was declared a panacea for cancer. The book became a bestseller, and hundreds of thousands of people ran out to buy this new, magical supplement. Coincidentally, one of the companies that made millions of dollars in profits from selling shark cartilage products was founded by William Lane's son, Andrew.

Those who promote "alternative" cancer therapies often accuse the medical community of colluding with pharmaceutical companies, but though we do sometimes see scandals break out in the pharmaceutical or academic world, we do not see such obvious "coincidences" like the Lanes promoting shark cartilage products. One could just ignore the moral aspect of this if the products actually helped, but many clinical trials involving products made out of shark cartilage have been carried out over the past decades, and not a single one of them has ever confirmed its supposedly miraculous properties. Lobbyists for this "alternative treatment" have long attempted to register their products as drugs, only to be repeatedly denied by the United States Food and Drug Administration due to their unproven effectiveness.

Unfortunately, this has not deterred them from selling their wares as a "dietary supplement," and unscrupulous individuals continue to profit from the desperation of patients and their families.

Not only does Lane's book rely on false content, but even the title is based on a fallacy. American ichthyologists, annoyed by the hype surrounding this snake oil, have proven that, in fact, sharks can get cancer, including cancer of the very cartilage tissue that the book attempts to promote as a panacea. Amusingly enough, there is one animal on earth that almost never gets cancer but thank goodness no one has thought of eating it yet (at least not on an industrial scale), though scientists around the world are actively studying it in laboratories.

It is the naked mole-rat (*Heterocephalus glaber*). Zoologists categorize naked mole-rats as rodents, but few laypeople would recognize these bald, blind animals with no ears (or at least, no outer ears) or the ability to maintain a constant body temperature as close relatives of hamsters or guinea pigs. The naked mole-rat is a burrowing animal with a massive (for its size) head and powerful jaws. Its lifestyle is even more unusual than its appearance.

The naked mole-rat lives in colonies that are similar in structure to the colonies of some social insects. Each of these groups is headed by a single female producer (the mother or queen), who mates with only two or three males. All of the other animals in the colony, whether they are male or female, are workers. Physiologically, they are capable of reproduction, though they do not reproduce themselves. As is the case in many social insects, if the queen is removed, several female workers will engage in a fierce battle to take her place.

What duties the worker naked mole-rats perform depends on their size. Small animals maintain the tunnel system, help take care of the young, and look for food (tubers). Larger workers act as "soldiers" and protect the colony from their main enemies — snakes. The queen is exclusively occupied with breeding, producing hundreds of young per year. All of this on its own would be enough to put this animal in a special category of the most unusual zoological curiosities, but their physiology and biochemistry are even more extraordinary. Naked mole-rats have a long lifespan, and can live up to thirty years, while the average lifespan of a similarly sized rodent is usually no longer than two or three years. Despite this incredible longevity, naked mole-rats only very rarely ever develop malignant tumors (a common disease among most rodents). For a long time, researchers believed that they were essentially cancer-free, but in 2016, an article was published about two cases of tumors that were recorded in a colony of naked mole-rats living in captivity. It raised a scientific sensation, though even these tumors grew unusually slowly compared to "typical" malignancy. Today, many laboratories around the world are studying naked mole-rats with the aim of understanding the secrets of aging and finding the key to curing cancer, hoping that perhaps some of the molecular mechanisms that protect this mammal from premature death can be used to benefit humans as well.

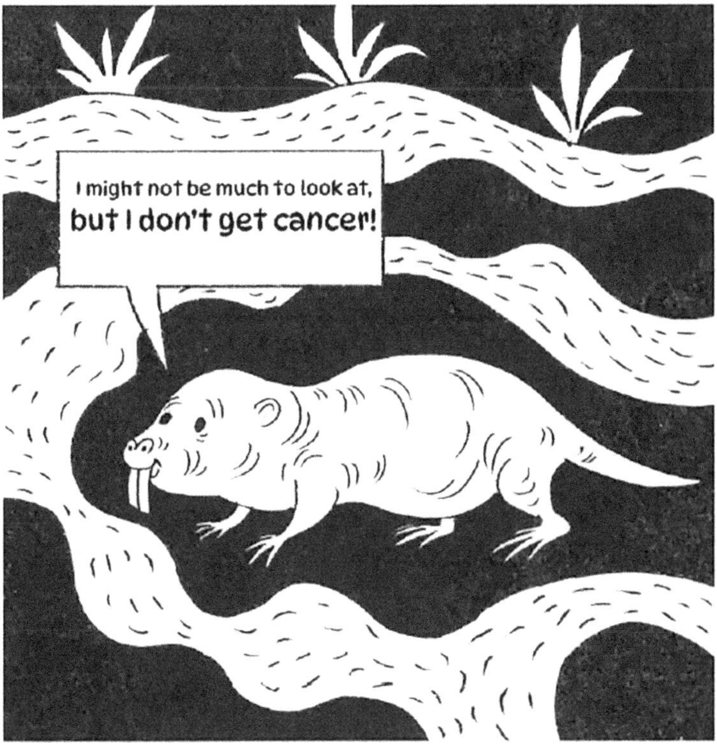
I might not be much to look at,
but I don't get cancer!

Figure 16. The naked mole-rat confirms – beauty is not the key to happiness! This African animal almost never gets cancer, and it also lives much longer than most of its closest relatives – rodents.

FACT: Nutritionists encourage you to regularly eat fish (wild caught rather than farm raised!) rather than any mythical shark cartilage. Indirect evidence shows that people who regularly eat fish are less likely to develop certain cancers.

SUMMARY

In this chapter, we learned about changes in cancer cell behavior, such as accelerated growth and frequent division, which go along with disruptions to energy metabolism, the foundation of cells' biomechanical economy. Cancer cells are greedy, and they wastefully consume glucose, oxidizing it only into lactic acid, rather than into carbon dioxide like a normal, healthy cell. This metabolic peculiarity is known as the Warburg effect, in honor of the first scientist who described the phenomenon. Scientists are currently trying to use the features of cancer cell metabolism to create new types of drugs and, so far, the Warburg effect is the basis for PET, which is one of the most accurate diagnostic methods available in oncology today. So far, we have discussed cancer cells and the cancerous tumor as a kind of entity in itself, though the tumor does not exist in a vacuum, but in a body. We also discussed how cancer cells interact with one another and the healthy tissue surrounding them. What is the "tumor microenvironment" and how does it influence tumor growth and metastasis? Why does the immune system not totally prevent the development of malignant tumors? Can we somehow "shake it up" and make it fight cancer more effectively? All of this is a topic for the next chapter.

Chapter 6
THE TUMOR ENVIRONMENT AND MYTHS ABOUT METASTASES

The main difference between malignant and benign tumors is not the speed of growth — many benign tumors also grow quickly and are capable of reaching rather impressive proportions — but the ability to spread throughout the body (metastasis) and produce new tumors in the most unexpected places.

This is the basis for classifying cancer stages — from stage one, when the tumor is localized in one place, to stage four, with multiple metastases throughout the body, and intermediate stages of occupying the surrounding lymph nodes and organs. Preventing this invasion is one of the key tasks of cancer treatment.

Unfortunately, as many patients do not see the doctor until they are already in the late stages (including due to their fears of being diagnosed with cancer), treatment often does not begin until the tumor is in active metastasis. That kind of timing led to the idea that tumors only begin to metastasize if you disturb them — through surgery or chemotherapy — but if you do not "bother" them, they will not metastasize. Of course, there are cases (not only with cancer) where treatment unfortunately will not only fail to cure the patient, but will even worsen their condition. But fortunately, cases like this are rare exceptions, while the spread of malignant cells throughout the body is a “rule”—the natural and inevitable progression of tumor growth.

In this chapter, we will discuss which factors determine cancer’s spread throughout the body and the role of cells in the tumor’s healthy “microenvironment.”

CANCEROUS RUBICON

In order to describe the process through which malignant tumors spread throughout the body, scientific literature uses two terms: "invasion" and "metastasis." It is not always easy to distinguish between them, but usually "invasion" is the term used when doctors observe tumors in the neighboring tissues and organs, while "metastasis" is used to describe the cancer's spread further throughout the body. There are two main paths to cancer's spread: one involves increased cell division, while the other is associated with the active migration of cancer cells.

In the first case, the tumor grows into the surrounding tissues, and simply pushes them apart and places pressure on them, like plants that begin to sprout and crack the sidewalk. When this type of growth enters the lymph nodes and blood vessels, the fluids begin to "wash away" additional cells or even fragments containing several cells, and the tumor begins to spread throughout the body. Thus, the invasion process is directly linked to the growth of new blood vessels within the tumor (angiogenesis). The more blood vessels, the greater the likelihood of metastasis.

In the second case, however, the cells or groups of cells that have broken away from the tumor actively move into the surrounding tissues, and once they reach a blood vessel, they can also spread throughout the body. That mobility of malignant cells is likely related to their ability to "rejuvenate," which we discussed in Chapter 4. Tumor cells are more similar to embryonic cells than mature ones, as fetal tissues are much more mobile than those of an adult organism. During the embryonic period, it is common for cells to "crawl" from place to place. Only later will tissues settle down and stay in one location.

In order to begin actively spreading throughout the body, cancer cells undergo what is known as the "epithelial–mesenchymal transition." In essence, the cell loses its properties as epithelial tissue (the main source of most cancerous tumors) and takes on the properties of mesenchymal tissue. Epithelial cells are characterized by their ability to form tight contact, and epithelial tissue is similar to a neatly arranged border — stone to stone, or rather, cell to cell, lasting and stable. Naturally, its main function in the human body is to act as a barrier. Mesenchymal cells, on the contrary, are mobile and capable of purposeful movement. In order to radically change its properties, the cell "cuts ties" with its neighbors and stops synthesizing E-cadherin proteins, which are responsible for forming tight contacts, and then rebuilds its cytoskeleton. The cytoskeleton fibers, which passively retain the shape of an epithelial cell, will be replaced with actin and vimentin fibers, which allow the cells to change shape and engage in purposeful movement.

It seems that both processes — spreading through proliferation (cell division) and migrating — take place in different tumors, or even in different places in the same tumor. Moreover, cancer cells can migrate and spread through division, either on their own or in "organized groups," which increases the chance of a successful invasion.

Recently, data has indicated that these two paths of metastasis are mutually exclusive. A cancer cell can either divide intensively or migrate rapidly, but it cannot do both at the same time. We cannot say that this is a particularly surprising observation. Both processes — migration and division — require rearranging the cell's inner skeleton. The same proteins form the "division spindle" during the M phase and form the bulges that make it possible for the cell to move around. It is possible that there simply is no configuration of the microtubule network that would allow cells to "divide on the way." However, the revelation of this obvious but previously unappreciated fact might have serious implications for adjusting cancer treatment. Many anti-tumor drugs are aimed at stopping cancer cell division. However, in some tumor models, their use can lead to a paradoxical (and extremely unpleasant) result, when the primary tumor is successfully suppressed, but suddenly many metastases appear. These types of pitfalls in traditional chemotherapy have led many oncologists to believe that an effective cancer treatment should aim to both decrease tumor growth and also prevent invasion via migration.

The study of cancer stem cells, which we discussed in Chapter 4, has suggested that a small but very active group of malignant cells is often responsible for cancer's spread throughout the body.

Scientists and doctors once believed that a tumor's ability to invade only comes about during the later stages of development. Generally speaking, this observation still holds true. A small tumor that is removed during the first or second stage is less likely to metastasize than a large neoplasm. However, unfortunately, there are exceptions to that rule. Some tumors seem to acquire the ability to metastasize even in the very earliest stages of development. It appears that this heightened malignancy is closely related to cancer cells' ability to loosen the intercellular matrix, which we will discuss later on. Additionally, there are cases as mentioned above in which the primary tumor disappears on its own, without a trace, having been defeated by the body's own defense mechanisms, but its "descendants"—the second generation of tumors formed via metastasis — continue to grow and spread through the patient's body. For this reason, no matter how successful the outlook appears after surgery, all cancer patients should be closely monitored for at least a few more years, in order to catch any potential return of the disease.

FACT: Invasion and metastasis are legitimate stages of cancer development.

CANCEROUS TUMORS AS BOTH SUPERPARASITES AND "EFFECTIVE MANAGERS"

Do internal factors alone, such as the speed of cellular division and/or the motility of cancer cells, influence whether a tumor will spread? Researchers are convinced that this is not the case. One of the most important breakthroughs in molecular oncology over the last decade has been the realization that cancer's "success" in the body is largely determined by the properties of the healthy tissues surrounding the tumor.

Sometimes, when we go to the theater to see a play, the supporting characters' reactions tell us all we need to know about the appearance of a main character. "The retinue makes the king," as they say in Russia. This is how a malignant tumor is "played" by its cellular environment. Over half of the cell mass in a pathological growth, a tumor, is in fact made up of healthy tissues — endothelial cells forming the thinnest vessels (capillaries), fibroblasts (connective tissue cells), lymphocytes, etc. Their behavior determines whether a tumor will grow and spread throughout the body, or if, on the contrary, the body's defenses will combine to destroy the malignant neoplasm.

The problem is that most cancerous tumors have highly enviable "leadership qualities." They are capable of sending special molecular signals to their external environment and taking over the cells in surrounding tissues, which are then forced to submit to the tumor's ever-growing needs. Researchers use the term "reprogramming" to highlight the depth of the changes that take place within normal cells affected by the tumor. Just like the members of a totalitarian religious cult, they lose themselves entirely and begin serving the malignant neoplasm instead.

Cancer's interaction with the body is eerily similar to that of a highly advanced parasite, which is so skilled at integrating into its host's life cycle that even at the brink of death the host will not notice what is happening. Carl Zimmer describes the "ideal parasite" in his book *Parasite Rex: Inside the Bizarre World of Nature's Most Dangerous Creatures*:[5]

> *The parasitic ideal was embodied by an unfortunate creature known as the Sacculina carcini. After hatching from an egg, the creature has a head, mouth, tail, legs, and a segmented body — everything that a crustacean should have. But rather than growing into a creature that would search for and source its own food, the sacculina simply finds a crab, attaches itself to it, and screws right onto its shell. Once inside the crab, the sacculina quickly degenerates, losing its segmented body, legs, tail, and even its mouth. Instead, it grows a rootlike antenna, which invades the crab's entire body. Having by this time degenerated into an almost plantlike state, it uses these antennae to suck nutrients from the crab.*

From a systems perspective, the *Sacculina* is as primitive as its host, as the tumor is more primitive than the organism that produced it. However, its ability to adapt to its conditions for existence (the crab's body) is almost perfect. The *Sacculina* does not only try to feed and grow at its host's expense. It changes its behavior so that the host begins to take care of the *Sacculina*'s larvae as if they were the crab's own young. This is how the cells surrounding a tumor are reprogrammed and allow not only the primary tumor to grow, but for cancer to spread throughout the body — metastasis. Vascular and connective tissue cells as well as immune cells, which we will touch on in the next chapter, are the main subjects of this reprogramming phenomenon.

---

[5] Carl Zimmer. Parasite Rex: Inside the Bizarre World of the World's Most Dangerous Creatures. (Chicago: Free Press, 2000).

FACT: Even healthy cells (free of cancerous mutations) in the tumor environment display pathological features.

MYSTERIES OF THE BLOOD – ANGIOGENESIS

German writer Erich Maria Remarque described the fluid flowing through our veins as "four liters of mystery and nonstop movement." For centuries and millennia, the image of blood has been inseparable from the image of life itself.

If a person lost blood and then died, they lost their life, and the blood in their body stopped flowing. In many religious traditions, blood was seen as something simultaneously sacred and "unclean." For example, the Old Testament states that "the soul of the body is in the blood," and therefore forbids eating the blood of animals that have been slaughtered (a dietary rule that is still followed by Jews and Muslims). Centuries before the discovery of hemoglobin, humankind was well aware of blood's significance.

Any healthy tissue needs a supply of nutrients and oxygen. In an organ (or part of an organ) with impaired blood circulation, the cells start dying off within a few minutes – this is why heart attacks and strokes can have such devastating consequences. Paradoxically, though, "diseased" cancer tissue requires an even more regular blood supply than healthy tissue. As we saw in the chapter on metabolism, cancer cells shift their metabolism to a more ancient, less effective pathway of biomechanical transformation, known as glycolysis. For this reason, cancer cells need to burn off more glucose than healthy cells to get the same amount of energy. They also need more oxygen – soon after the tumor begins to grow, there will appear to be areas that are suffering from an oxygen deficit, "hypoxia," and the tumor's fate depends on whether or not it is able to increase its cell mass at the same time as building its vascular growth in order to ensure it receives sufficient nutrition and aeration.

The thinnest blood vessels of the cardiovascular system — the capillaries — are formed by a layer of thick endothelial cells surrounded by a dense basal membrane of protein fibers, forming a delicate tube that is soft inside, but rigid on the outside. The tumor cells, which lack oxygen, will begin to actively produce two types of protein: proteases, which can break down the basal membrane, and special growth factors that stimulate vascular growth. The most important and well-studied of these growth factors are vascular endothelial growth factor (VEGF) proteins. The proteases "eat holes" in the protein-impermeable basal membrane, and the growth factors are able to reach the exposed endothelial cells, bind to the corresponding receptors, and transmit a signal to increase the vascular network.

In response, the endothelial cells begin to divide and grow in the direction of the signal source, forming a sort of outgrowth from the existing blood vessel, much in the same way that plant roots grow in the same direction as moisture and nutrients; the capillary branching system even looks like a tangle of thin roots. This is how the tumor is able to encourage blood vessels to grow in its direction and provide it with a supply of oxygen and nutrients, along with the ability to metastasize.

After studying the mechanisms for tumor angiogenesis, scientists hypothesized that disrupting this process might slow down tumor growth, and possibly destroy the tumor entirely. If the tumor is deprived of nutrients and especially oxygen, it should simply die, just as brain or heart tissue does during a stroke or heart attack. Could that be the silver bullet that cures several types of cancer at once? Researchers have enthusiastically tested many potential angiogenesis inhibitors. Currently, several drugs that block VEGF signaling pathways have been approved for clinical use, such as bevacizumab (Avastin). Unfortunately, there was no miracle here — not one of these drugs can entirely halt the vascular growth process, as researchers had hoped. VEGF is the main factor for angiogenesis, but it is not the only signaling protein directing this process. It is likely that other growth factor proteins are at least partially capable of compensating for a lack of VEGF in the tumor. However, when combined with other agents, anti-VEGF therapy has shown itself to be highly effective at treating some types of cancer, such as kidney cancer. Researchers continue to study the molecular mechanisms behind vascular growth in search of less obvious but possibly more effective molecular targets for the development of new drugs.

FACT: The substances that inhibit angiogenesis are present in green tea, tomatoes, soy products, etc. For this reason, some scientists believe that these foods should be part of any "anti-cancer diet." Others believe that this kind of dietary approach has never been proven effective, though they see no harm in regularly consuming those foods.

Seek, and ye shall find

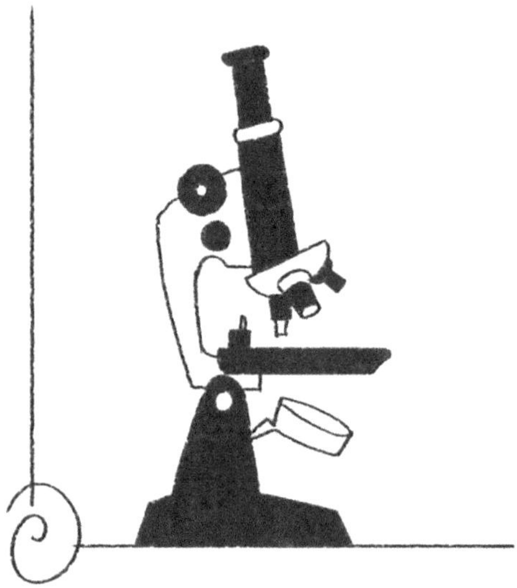

As much as we want to believe that medicine in general and pharmacology in particular develop in neat, sequential series of well-planned steps and conclusions, we have to admit that there have been, and continue to be, an astonishing number of unpredictable "happy accidents." Fleming discovered penicillin by accident; studying the chemical warfare agent we know as mustard gas led to the advent of chemotherapy; Viagra was initially developed as a heart disease drug and certainly not for the purpose of maintaining an erection — and these are just some of the more colorful examples.

There is another story like this related to the "side effects" of anti-angiogenic drugs. Anti-VEGF therapy, which was developed for treating malignant tumors, and which did not entirely fulfill scientists' expectations, turned out to be a highly effective drug for an entirely different disease. Cancer is not the only disease that involves pathological angiogenesis. Many elderly people suffer from excessive vascular growth in the retina, in a condition known as age-related macular degeneration. This disease often causes blindness in seniors, which significantly worsens their quality of life. Previously, treatment involved many complex manipulations, with no results guaranteed. Now, in most cases, the disorder can be cured with literally just a few injections of anti-angiogenic drugs. This is a classic example of how in biology, if you look long enough and deep enough, you are sure to run into something, albeit not necessarily what you were looking for when you started.

OUR SECOND SKELETON

The intercellular matrix plays a key role in a tumor's spread, no matter which way it goes. When we talk about the cellular structure of the human body, we are usually imagining dense rows of cells, stacked together like bricks in a wall. In fact, though, in most of our body's tissues, with the exception of muscle and epithelial cells, the cells are arranged rather loosely. The intercellular matrix is what "glues" them together so that the body can function as a unit.

Unlike plant and bacterial cells, which have a dense cell wall, human cells are soft sacs filled with cytoplasm, which is why we do not just puddle onto the floor, and instead maintain the density and elasticity of the tissues that shape our body. We have the extracellular matrix to thank for this ability. Structurally, we might even consider this to be our "second skeleton." Under a microscope, the matrix looks like a dense network of fibers braiding cells together, and the space between them is filled with extracellular fluid.

Collagen is the extracellular matrix's main structural protein (more specifically, collagens, which are a group of proteins). Collagen provides cells with structural support and makes tissues hard and resistant. Its partner, the protein elastin, is no less important, and makes tissues more elastic and stretchy, so we find it wherever that is most needed (for example in the ligaments and artery walls). The balance between collagen and elastin fibers will determine any given tissue's or organ's main mechanical properties, but there are also many other biomolecules in the matrix.

Many extracellular matrix proteins are strongly glycosylated, which means that their amino acids form a chemical bond with various carbohydrates (sugars). The weight of carbohydrates in a mature molecule of these proteins can make up 90 to 95 percent of the protein, while the share of amino acid residues will be just 5 to 10 percent. These proteins are known as proteoglycans, and due to the many

OH-groups in sugars, they are able to retain water and other biologically active substances, much like a sponge.

The most important non-protein component of the matrix is hyaluronic acid, which is known for its unique ability to bind a large number of water molecules. Hyaluronic acid is widely used in cosmetology as a nourishing cream or injection to fill in wrinkles.

The extracellular matrix is very active as it interacts with the cells that are immersed in it. Proteins — collagens and fibronectins — bind to membrane proteins known as integrins, and give the cell various signals to stop dividing, begin moving, or even die. This dynamic is constantly renewing the structure, as special enzymes (matrix metalloproteinases) carry out regular "cleanups" in the collagen "forest," and new matrix components are synthesized in fibroblasts to replace the old ones.

In a malignant tumor, that normal structure of the extracellular matrix is disrupted. It becomes looser, stops holding the cells together, and limits their ability to divide. It is this change in properties in the extracellular matrix that largely distinguishes a malignant tumor from a benign one and gives malignant cells the ability to metastasize. Of course, these changes do not simply happen out of nowhere. In order to modify the environment to best serve their needs, the cells will take over the connective tissue cells — fibroblasts.

Normally, fibroblasts function to control the state of the extracellular matrix, break down old collagen and elastin fibers (proteins also age), and synthesize new ones. In cancer, however, these cells are "reprogrammed" by the tumor so that they serve its needs — the cancer cells literally "tame" the fibroblasts by secreting special substances in order to later use them as "cash cows." When the connective tissue cells submit to the tumor, they begin secreting valuable nutrients into their environment, such as glutamate and ketone bodies, literally "feeding" their malignant neighbors. As fibroblasts abandon their normal functions, they produce more growth factors that stimulate cancer cell division and the growth of new blood vessels, so that once the tumor has grown enough, it is able to spread throughout the body.

Scientists have discovered that fibroblasts act as a sort of "guide" for cancer cells, paving the way for them in the collagen matrix, much as the first skier walking on the snowy ground paves the way for those behind them. But in this case, the followers are migrating cancer cells, which will follow fibroblasts not only one by one, but in whole colonies. The tumor fibroblasts are the main source of the TGF⊠ protein, which activates cancer cells' epithelial–mesenchymal transition, through which they acquire motility. This is how help in various forms from healthy, non-transformed cells contributes to cancer's spread through the body.

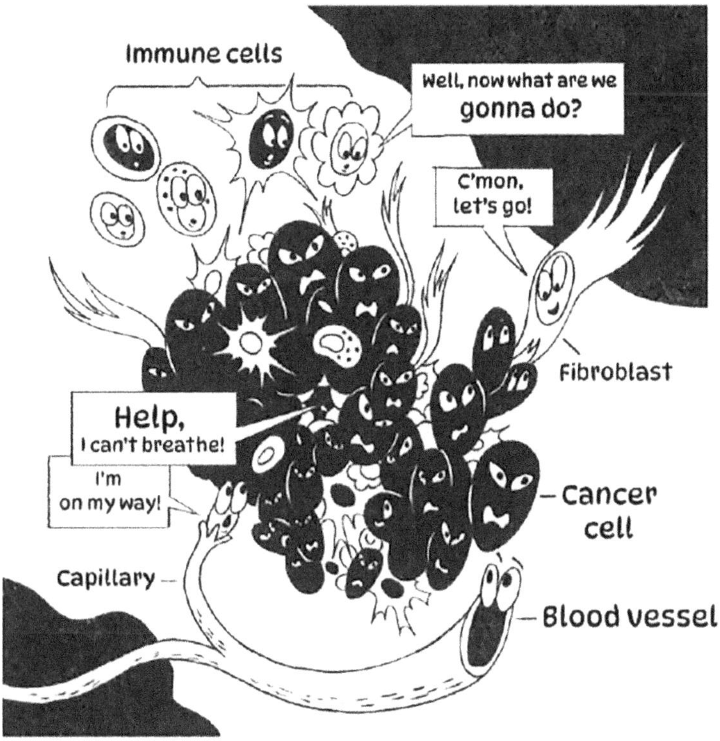

Figure 17. A tumor's microenvironment will determine the speed at which it grows and spreads through the body. Blood vessels growing into the tumor will supply cancer cells with nutrients and oxygen, while fibroblasts will facilitate metastasis. This is how the tumor's microenvironment is associated with several key features of cancer (see Figure 1).

FACT: As we age, the number of fibroblasts in our body decreases, and the process for renewing the extracellular matrix slows down, although that happens at different speeds in different tissues. In the last several years, one beauty trend has involved injecting the client's own fibroblasts into "problem areas" of her (usually it is a her) face, in order to activate the synthesis of necessary substances there. However, before deciding to take the leap and attempt this procedure, you should be aware that the long-term consequences of this therapy (including the development of cancerous tumors) have not been well researched.

A WOUND THAT WILL NOT HEAL

Why are normal cells so willing to carry out a tumor's "molecular orders"? The answer lies in the fact that the tumor's behavior mimics the normal processes that take place in the body when regenerating damaged tissues. Because of this similarity, oncologist Harold Dvorak entitled his 1986 article "Tumors: Wounds That Do Not Heal." When we are dealing with a real injury like a cut or fracture, growing blood vessels, supplying nutrients, and speeding up cellular division are good things. Unfortunately, in the case of a tumor, these processes will not lead to healing, but the patient's condition getting worse. "Reprogramming" healthy cells in the tumor's environment is an important factor in cancer development, and this creates a state of chronic inflammation, which goes hand in hand with a "wound that will not heal."

In a healthy body, inflammation is a normal defense mechanism that is part of a response to mechanical or infectious tissue damage. It manifests as a set of physical reactions aimed at removing damaging products or agents and restoring integrity to the area. This condition was described by ancient physicians Celsus and Galen, and is well known to anyone who has ever suffered from an acute respiratory infection or gotten a splinter:

- redness (localized, of the skin or mucosa)
- swelling (edema)
- fever (an increase in local temperature)
- pain
- dysfunction.

At the organism level, this is what inflammation looks like. If we were to try to observe the process in molecular detail, however, we would see the following picture: The destruction of cells leads to their contents spilling out into the extracellular environment, thus sending a "Danger!" signal to the surrounding tissue. This causes the metabolism in the injured area to be restructured. Consumption of both glucose and oxygen increases at the same time (this is why, as we described in Chapter 5, PET scans often cannot distinguish between tumors and inflammation). As a result of the metabolic changes, lactic acid begins to accumulate in the area, which becomes "acidic" (just like the tumor) as inflammation begins. Blood vessels at the site of the injury will dilate and increase blood flow, as the blood flow itself slows down, which causes redness and a localized temperature increase. The walls of the small blood vessels — capillaries — become more permeable, which leads to the release of immune cells and the liquid part of blood (plasma) at the site of the injury — this is how an edema is formed, which squeezes the nerve endings, causing pain.

After the immune system cells destroy the damaging factors and "eat" the destroyed cells, which cleanses the wound, fibroblasts begin restoring the intracellular matrix (scarring), and the inflammation usually subsides quickly. This inflammatory reaction, which is fast and passes with minimal consequences, is called "acute" or "subacute" (depending on its duration). Unfortunately, an untreated infection or allergy sometimes does not entirely disappear, but remains in the body as so-called chronic inflammation. Chronic inflammation is much less bothersome than acute, as all of the symptoms are more subdued — the pain is not severe, the swelling is moderate. That is both good (it is less bothersome for the patient) and bad. If the patient does not pay more attention to it, this kind of pathological process can become the basis for more serious diseases — including the development of cancer, as the factors supporting inflammation also lead to DNA damage.

Many cancers follow advanced inflammatory processes. Stomach cancer often develops in cases of gastritis or ulcers, and colon cancer usually takes place after local inflammation (colitis), and of course the main cause of liver cancer is cirrhosis, caused by hepatitis.

In light of growing evidence on the relationship between inflammation and malignant degeneration, scientists have turned their attention to traditional, well-studied anti-inflammatory drugs. After all — should they not have cancer-fighting properties too? A few decades ago, doctors discovered that the classic anti-inflammatory drug, aspirin, can help prevent the development of cardiovascular diseases, including heart attacks, if taken regularly. Given the low cost of this treatment, the well-studied and minor side effects, and the enormous benefit potential, many primary care doctors in both the United States and Europe have begun prescribing aspirin to their elderly patients, en masse. Over the decades, researchers have gathered a large body of statistics on people who regularly take aspirin (a daily dose is lower than what we take for aches and pains). Doctors studied the figures and compared people who regularly take aspirin to those who do not, and discovered that not only does aspirin prevent cardiovascular disease, it also lowers the likelihood of developing tumors in the digestive system by 15 to 20 percent. The results for colon cancer — which is one of the most common cancers among elderly people — were particularly surprising. Currently, researchers are studying the potential of aspirin and other anti-inflammatory drugs to lower the risk of other types of cancer.

Scientists continue to debate the molecular mechanisms behind inflammation's influence on cancer development, but some practical conclusions are already obvious to the experts — timely elimination of any source of chronic inflammation, no matter how trivial it may seem, lowers one's risk of developing malignant neoplasms in that location. The cost of these preventive measures is a fraction of the material and moral cost of treating a cancerous tumor, but it does require all of us to be attentive and responsible when it comes to our health.

The moral of the story: as we wait for new scientific miracles, do not lose sight of good old prevention — get regular check-ups with your primary care doctor and gastroenterologist, gynecologist, or urologist, and take care of infections right away. It may seem boring and uninspiring, like taking a daily aspirin (consult your physician first!), but it can add years to your life, and make what time you have much more valuable.

FACT: Chronic inflammation in any part of the body is a risk factor that can trigger malignant transformation.

FIND YOUR NICHE

For some time, doctors have known that cancer's spread throughout the body is not a random process. Cancer cells of various origins metastasize, and as a rule, to certain organs, and sometimes even in a specific sequence. Breast cancer, for example, will first metastasize to the bones, liver, lymph nodes, lungs, and then the brain. This pattern is known as "organotropic metastasis." How do we explain this apparent selectivity?

Leaving the tumor in order to travel freely throughout the body is only half the battle for a cancer cell. Of the tumor cells that manage to enter the bloodstream each day, less than 1 percent will actually survive and have a chance of producing distant metastases. For a secondary tumor to form, a cell must detach and then successfully take root in another part of the body, which will have a completely different, unfamiliar microenvironment.

As early as 1889, English surgeon Stephen Paget, who is considered the founder of modern metastatic theory, compared the spread of metastases to the spread of seeds that scatter in all possible directions, but only germinate where they have found the right soil. However, exactly what factors determine the order of tumor colonization in the body, and why some organs turn out to be more suitable for some cancers, while others attract different cancers, remained a mystery for a very long time.

Initially, it was assumed that tumors spread solely based on the general layout of the circulatory system. If blood passed through organ A, which had a malignant tumor, and then moved toward organ B, it was only logical to assume that most metastases would settle there. During the 1970s, however, an experiment shed doubt on this very simple explanation.

The experiment, like most involving tumor transfer, used "nude mice." These are a special laboratory breed of mice, which have a gene mutation that makes their immune system so underdeveloped that they can be transplanted with tumor fragments from other mice or even humans, and the tumor will not be rejected. Researchers injected radioactively labeled melanoma cells into the mice's bloodstreams, and then observed them. It turned out that though the cancer cells initially stopped in the liver and lungs, they formed secondary tumors only in the lungs, and did not survive in the liver. It became clear that the ability to colonize an organ depends on the direction of the blood flow as well as on the properties of the cancer cells themselves.

Further experiments revealed that the primary tumor lays the groundwork for future metastases by facilitating the formation of so-called pre-metastatic niches. Cancer cells produce a variety of biologically active substances that spread around the entire body through the blood flow, and determine the tumor type's ability to colonize various tissues.

In order to prove this, researchers conducted a rather elegant experiment using Lewis lung carcinoma cells. This type of cancer is unique in that, in the mice, it only metastasized to the lungs, and not to any other organs. However, if prior to being injected with the Lewis carcinoma cells the mice were injected with the liquid in which the melanoma cells were grown (just the liquid, without any cancer cells), things changed. The Lewis carcinoma cells began forming metastases in the organs where melanoma tends to metastasize (that is, the kidneys, spleen, etc.).

A study of tumors' secretion mechanisms showed that small membrane vesicles are most responsible for a tumor's long-range influence on the body. These vesicles contain biologically active substances that are carried through the body via the blood flow and release their contents in certain organs, which prepares them for future metastases. The vesicles spread various factors, such as VEGF and TGF⊠, which we already know as well as CCL2, a cytokine. CCL2 facilitates tumor spread by inhibiting local immunity in the vicinity of the pre-metastatic niche and prevents lymphocytes from efficiently destroying metastases.

Today, many laboratories are searching for a way to prevent the formation of pre-metastatic niches. If they succeed, it would be as significant as the discovery of retroviral therapy for AIDS treatment. Though that treatment is not capable of fully ridding the body of immunodeficiency virus, it keeps the infection under control and makes it possible for people with HIV to live full lives for decades. In the same way, making it possible to control cancer's metastasis would help control its malignancy and significantly lower cancer death rates. For now, however, such a radical solution is still just a dream.

One reason why it is so difficult to control metastases with drugs is the fact that it is a complicated process involving several different types of cells and signaling pathways at once. Nonetheless, scientists have seen some success in this area. Many tumors involve the c-Met protein, a receptor for hepatocyte growth factor (HGF). Strengthening signals that pass through that receptor increases cell motility and cancer's ability to metastasize.

Blocking HGF/c-MET pathway signals in a tumor addresses several issues at once. On one hand, it lowers cancer cells' motility, while also inhibiting vascular growth, since HGF is an angiogenic factor, just like VEGF proteins. Finally, the HGF/c-MET signal pathway is one of the main pathways for fibroblast "reprogramming," which means that inhibiting it also makes it possible to improve the tumor microenvironment. This complex effect on the tumor and its environment simultaneously blocks that pathway and is particularly effective at preventing the spread of tumors with an active c-MET oncogene. There are several anti-HGF therapy drugs already on the market, such as cabozantinib and crizotinib, while others are still in clinical trials.

FACT: Metastases that have been lying dormant in metastatic niches can "awaken" and make themselves known several years after the primary tumor has been successfully treated, which is why it takes several years after the completion of therapy to talk about being "cancer-free."

SUMMARY

In this chapter, we learned that cancer cells are capable of "reprogramming" normal, healthy cells in the human body and, just like a highly specialized parasite, forcing them to serve it. Malignant tumors imitate the behavior of a "wound that will not heal," which the body will try to heal by growing new blood vessels into it and providing it with nutrients. Spreading throughout the body, or metastasis, is a natural consequence of tumor growth and changes to the tumor cells' properties as a result of epithelial–mesenchymal transition. This takes place when detached cells spread through the body, using special pre-metastatic niches formed in the organs vulnerable to the biologically active substances produced by the primary tumor.

What about the immune system? Why is it incapable or unwilling to protect the body from disease? In the next chapter, we will discuss tumors' ability to deceive the body's natural immune system, along with new methods for strengthening anti-cancer immune response.

Chapter 7
THE FINER POINTS OF IDENTIFYING "THE OTHER" AND MYTHS ABOUT IMMUNITY

Immunology is a fascinating field that has been practiced for centuries (vaccinations, blood group selection during transfusions, etc.) and it is a full-fledged scientific foundation for the body's mechanisms for identifying friend or foe.

The general public's attitude toward immunology varies between complete denial (as we see in the "anti-vax" movement and the HIV-denial community that does not believe in the existence of the AIDS virus) to quasi-religious belief in the body's own defenses—"Just strengthen your immune system!"

As usual, the truth is far from either extreme. The immune system does play an important role in preventing cancerous tumors, and there are ways to enhance its ability to recognize and destroy cancer cells, but we have yet to come close to making immunotherapy the primary method for fighting cancer.

There are some local and general immune stimulation methods that work very well on certain types of tumors. Unfortunately, not every patient has a chance to receive treatment with the latest immunotherapy drugs, as it is very expensive, though there is hope that in time that will change. On the other hand, there are also inventors of various types of quackery promising "natural immunity enhancement" and 100 percent recovery as they ride the information wave that followed announcements of immunotherapy successes.

What mechanisms does our immune system use to fight off disease? Why are some tumors more sensitive to immune response than others? Are there cases of tumors spontaneously healing, or is that just folklore? In this chapter, we will discuss the strengths and weaknesses of our body's defenses.

SPONTANEOUS REMISSION – A MIRACLE YOU CANNOT COUNT ON

There is no shortage of videos out there with people talking about all sorts of miracle cures for cancer, claiming to speak "from my own experience"—"I was sick, in stage three or four, nothing was helping, and I started taking XXX, and within just a few months I was cured!" Some of these people are probably just shamelessly lying, but there is always the possibility that some of them are telling the truth about their disease and some miracle cure, though the cure actually has nothing to do with consuming baking soda or any sort of magical mushrooms. Spontaneous cancer recovery is a rare but consistently observed phenomenon, though its occurrence after the use of any "alternative treatment" is probably just a coincidence. Another example of this is the "survivor error," when we hear about the one person who took a miracle drug and recovered, but we do not hear about the widespread "silent testimonies" of the many other patients who were less fortunate and died.

In the next chapter, on evidence-based medicine, we will talk about why the claims of "I tried it and it worked!" should probably not be believed. However, the phenomenon of spontaneous remission from cancer shows that our bodies do have forces capable of beating the disease on its own in certain conditions. Naturally, that phenomenon is of great interest to scientists.

The likelihood of spontaneous healing depends on the type of tumor. In some diseases, like kidney cancer and melanoma, it is more frequent; in others, it is rarer. In some types of brain cancers, known as neuroblastomas, which are most frequent in infants, the rate of spontaneous remission is so high that, in some cases, doctors prefer to delay treatment. In fact, in children under one year of age, the chances of spontaneous healing are higher than the likelihood of a successful medical intervention.

Because of the low probability of spontaneous remission, though, it is difficult to conduct a systematic study, and we do not yet have a detailed description of its mechanisms. However, there is no doubt that activating the immune response plays a major role in the body's ability to beat cancer. This can be caused by changes in the tumor properties that take place as it evolves, or external events which at first glance appear unrelated to the disease. For example, while researching statistics on spontaneous remission from leukemia, scientists discovered that in 90 percent of the cases, the patients healed following a severe infection, such as pneumonia. It seems that the body's general mobilization of its defenses against a microbial invasion can also lead to victory over the tumor. What an example of "whatever does not kill us makes us stronger"!

FACT: There are some cases in which the patient's body is able to defeat cancer on its own, but the likelihood of spontaneous remission is about the same as winning the lottery jackpot — about one in one hundred thousand.

GERMS AS CANCER FIGHTERS

It is interesting to note that ancient physicians were already considering ways to treat cancer by activating the body's own defenses, thousands of years before scientists had come up with the term "immunity."

An ancient Egyptian manuscript by Imhotep (2600 BC) talked about healing "swellings" (presumably cancerous tumors) with an infection in the same organ. In the nineteenth century, these cases were the first officially documented by doctors. Prior to the advent of antibiotics, it was common for wounds to get infected. Observant doctors had noticed that if inflammation or gaseous gangrene appeared in the same location as the tumor they had just operated on, the cancer was much less likely to recur. Often, the recovery was complete. Unfortunately, at the time, it was impossible to control the progression of such infections, and there was always the risk that gangrene would destroy the tumor but then kill the patient. This risk was simply too high to suggest that these observations should be used for any therapeutic treatment.

It was nearly a hundred years until, in the early twentieth century, American doctor William Kohli proposed his own microbial cancer treatment, which became the first type of immunotherapy. Kohli injected a "cocktail" of weakened bacteria that he had developed into a postoperative wound. The mixture caused a sufficiently acute inflammatory reaction at the injection site, without killing the patient. Kohli used his method to treat inoperable sarcomas and managed to partially and even completely cure many patients, which by today's standards is impressive success for this type of tumor.

Unfortunately, Kohli's research was forgotten after his death, but fifty years later, there is a new wave of developments in immunological science, and the idea of enlisting the help of controlled infections to treat cancer is once again relevant. The result has been the first officially registered bacterial agent for cancer treatment.

This drug was initially designed to treat superficial forms of bladder cancer, and is made from a mixture of BCG (bacillus Calmette–Guérin) bacteria — the very same kind that we find in the tuberculosis vaccine. Weakened bovine tubercle bacillus (*Mycobacterium bovis* BCG) does not cause disease in humans, but it is capable of activating our immune response against tuberculosis and tumor cells. As a vaccine against tuberculosis, BCG is used intramuscularly, but when used to prevent complications from bladder cancer, it is injected into a cavity in the affected organ several weeks after surgery.

The drug's molecular mechanisms of action are not entirely clear, but it is obvious that there is some sort of local immune response activation. In any case, this medication can lower the risk of cancer relapse by several times, with far fewer side effects than most forms of traditional chemotherapy.

For decades, scientists have been searching for cancer drugs, showing time and again the wonders of inventiveness and intuition, though in the last several years, oncologists have concluded that definitive victory over the disease cannot be achieved without activating the body's own forces. Understanding the nuances of the immune response in cancer and seeking ways to strengthen it are the main tasks of the young but quickly developing science of oncoimmunology.

FACT: Mobilization of the immune response during an infection can in some cases lead to a pronounced anti-cancer effect.

TWO IMMUNE RESPONSES

Just as a wise army commander uses different types of troops to achieve a common goal — beating the enemy — the body uses various types of immune cells, often referred to together as "leukocytes" (white blood cells; as opposed to red blood cells, also known as erythrocytes) to defend itself. We can distinguish two main "divisions" from the immune system "army"—innate immune cells (macrophages, dendritic cells, natural killer cells) and acquired immune cells (lymphocytes).

Innate immune cells are fast, but not particularly selective, while acquired immune cells form more slowly, but are more effective due to their ability to "remember an enemy's face." By interacting and mutually reinforcing one another, these cells are capable of effectively counteracting most of the dangers threatening our bodies.

Immune cells' main talent is the ability to recognize antigens, or the "biological bodies and molecules carrying signs of foreign biological information." [6] The main antigens are proteins, though some bacterial polysaccharides and lipids are also capable of provoking a protective reaction in the human body.

If we were to compare the immune system to a medical care system, the innate immunity is like the ambulance we call when there is an obvious threat to the body, when there are symptoms such as loss of consciousness, high fever, and acute pain. The ambulance's job is to provide emergency care and give the body a chance to survive until it can be treated by specialists — acquired immune cells.

When a leukocyte detects a cell marked with foreign antigens, it first tries to destroy it on its own, and then "calls for help," sending special signaling molecules into its environment so that other immune

---

[6] Ярилин А.А. Иммунология. — М.: ГЭОТАР-Медиа, 2010. С. 264. (In Russian).

cells come to its aid. These active substances — cytokines and chemokines — trigger immune cell activity and are very important for the formation of a complete immune response.

The intensity of the immune reaction depends on the number of antigens and the quality of their recognition (binding strength). The more molecules the immune cell recognizes on the surface of the suspected foreign body, the stronger and more effective the response will be.

Molecules that induce an anti-cancer immune response are known as tumor antigens. These include proteins that have mutated within tumors (including due to the incorporation of oncoviruses into their genes) and the oncofetal antigens that we are already familiar with — embryonic proteins that begin synthesizing as a result of cancer cells' "rejuvenation." Normally, these macromolecules are only produced during the early stages of embryonic development, when immunity is not yet active, and so they are unfamiliar to the immune system of the adult organism and therefore perceived as foreign.

Recognizing an antigen, whether it is a tumor, viral, or bacterial, begins with the development of an immune response. The goal is to destroy the source of the foreignness and restore genetic unity and the organism's integrity.

FACT: Both innate and acquired immune responses are important for recognizing and destroying cancer cells.

KNOW THINE ENEMY

Macrophages, the main innate immune cells, are like large, eternally ravenous amoebas. In infectious invasions, they are the first to arrive at the place of infection, usually within minutes, and are capable of holding back pathological process development by eating viruses, bacteria, and other "suspicious" cells until the body's main defensive forces are mobilized.

Macrophages recognize "typical" bacterial and viral molecules, like polysaccharides in bacterial cell walls, and also react to any violent destruction of cells. As we described in the chapter on inflammation, this goes along with the release of special "horror molecules," which signal danger. To describe innate immune cells' recognition mechanism, scientists have introduced the poetic definition of "pathogenicity image." In essence, innate immune cells recognize not specific bacteria, but molecules that are common to many of them. Without getting into details, that means a certain average "bacterial infection" and general "destruction of cells."

Unlike those rapid response forces, T-cells, the adaptive immune system's main workhorses, need to adjust to each new pathogen (viral, bacterial, tumor). This process takes some time, and the immune response develops rather slowly — over a few days. However, once they have been activated against a certain enemy, the adaptive immune system retains that memory for a long time (sometimes forever), and next time, it will nip the disease in the bud. This secondary immune response against familiar infections develops so quickly that the disease does not usually even have time to manifest any symptoms.

This feature of the adaptive immune system (slow primary response and rapid secondary response) explains why children in daycares and elementary schools fall ill far more often than their parents, with all kinds of upper respiratory infections. The parents' bodies are already familiar with most viruses circulating in the area and capable of thwarting them, while the child's body is still getting to know them and developing a primary response.

Prophylactic vaccinations work on the basis of immune cells' immune memory effect, including those against tumors caused by viruses. By training the immune system in advance to recognize a killed or weakened form of the microbe, we are able to achieve a rapid, effective response to that infection in the future.

Though "training" is the most common metaphor used to describe activation of the immune response, it is not quite correct. In fact, the T-cells best suited for fighting a certain enemy are targeted out of their millions of counterparts. One can imagine a sort of molecular casting call, in order to find out "who here is best at recognizing this antigen and binding to it most strongly."

The main molecule responsible for recognizing foreign antigens is the T-cell receptor (TCR), which consists of immunoglobulin proteins. This group of proteins has a unique gene feature, which is the presence of special hypervariable sites that actively mutate and reshuffle within the T-cells. As a result, many different types of receptors are read from the same gene in different T-cells. Due to their diversity, these TCR hypervariable sites are responsible for recognizing foreign proteins (more specifically, foreign peptides).

The TCR molecules' "friend or foe" recognition system is very simple and also wasteful at once. (However, more than one generation of twentieth-century immunologists has racked their brains trying to understand this "simplicity.") While developing *in utero*, the human embryo forms cells that are precursors to T-cells, known as thymocytes, within a special organ called the thymus. Thymocytes synthesize an incredible variety of TCR subunits capable of recognizing any imaginable or even unimaginable amino acid sequence. The organism then tests these cells, which are not yet mature, for their ability to recognize (bind to) common proteins in the body (specifically, peptides, but we'll elaborate more on that later). The progenitor cells that have corresponding TCR variants on their surfaces are ruthlessly destroyed. This is how the immune system develops a tolerance to the body's own proteins, and the T-cells that carry a huge repertoire of various receptors, but only to alien antigens, undergo selection.

Different T-cells carry different sets of TCRs, which is why it takes time to find the cells among them that are most suitable for recognizing specific foreign proteins. This (among other things) explains the delay in adaptive immune response versus the innate one.

The T-cells that have been selected to bind a suitable antigen begin to divide intensely. As a result, several active lymphocytes form an entire army of clones ready to attack the enemy. And then, just like in an epic Hollywood blockbuster, a new superhero, lymphocyte, takes the place of any fighter lost in battle!

FACT: The presence of a large number of active T-cells in a tumor is a good sign for the patient's outlook and indicates a high likelihood of a successful cure.

ANTIGENS AND ANTIBODIES

The second important group of adaptive immune cells is B-cells, also known as B-lymphocytes, which are also capable of targeting antigens due to B-cell receptors, which are a close molecular relative to TCRs. Unlike TCRs, however, which are always bound to the cell membrane, there are two forms of B-cell receptors: membrane-bound or water-soluble. The water-soluble form, capable of recognizing a specific antigen, is called an antibody.

B-cells are activated in much the same way as T-cells, though they do not directly attack the enemy. Instead, B-cells react to the presence of a foreign antigen by producing antibodies to it. Those antibodies "stick" to the surface of bacterial or cancer cells and send a signal to other immune system cells: "This is an enemy, and it must be destroyed." B-cells can be compared to strict factory inspectors who check items coming off the assembly line, marking those with defects to be scrapped.

The role of natural B-cell immunity in the body's fight against cancer is not yet fully understood, but without the use of antibodies, we cannot imagine modern medicine or, for that matter, modern molecular biology. Their ability to selectively bind to certain proteins is used in diagnostics, such as pregnancy tests and certain therapies.

In order to obtain antibodies for human proteins in laboratories, scientists usually use B-cells from mice. The mice are injected with a serum containing macromolecules for which it is necessary to obtain antibodies (that is, to actually "inoculate" with human proteins rather than just viral or bacterial proteins), and then active B-cells producing the antibody to this antigen are isolated from the blood. However, direct use of the B-cells is restricted by the mice's "Hayflick limit." These are cells that also age and die over time. In order to obtain the necessary antibodies on an industrial scale, scientists had to develop hybridoma technology.

If two cells are placed next to one another and subjected to a substance that partially disrupts the cell membrane structure, they will fuse into one, just as two water droplets that touch each other will merge into one large droplet. By merging B-cells to malignant plasmacytoma cells this way, scientists have managed to obtain an immortal, high-performance source of antibodies. (When B-cells and plasmacytoma cells fuse, they form binuclear hybrids, but during subsequent divisions, the chromosomes of both cells will mix and form a single nucleus. This is how true hybrids, or hybridomas, are formed, which is where we get the name for the method, "hybridoma technology.")

There may be several different antibodies for one antigen (foreign protein) in the body, and they will bind to different parts of it. At the same time, each individual B-cell (and its descendants) only produces one kind of monoclonal antibody, that is, identical copies of one antibody.

In 1984, scientists Georges Köhler, César Milstein, and Niels Jerne won the Nobel Prize for their work developing hybridoma technology to produce monoclonal antibodies. They were offered a patent for their discovery, a decision which would have certainly made them millionaires (if not billionaires), given the extremely high demand for the new method. But as a true scientist, Milstein refused to profit from the results of scientific research, preferring to make the cutting-edge technology available to all biologists and physicians around the world, in order to serve humanity as a whole rather than the interests of a handful of individuals and corporations.

When antibodies are used as a medication, their name always ends in "-mab," which comes from "monoclonal antibody." Many new generation anti-cancer drugs mentioned in this book are part of that group, such as trastuzumab, which contains monoclonal antibodies that block the *HER2* receptor.

FACT: Antibodies in mice are capable of inducing an immune response in humans. In 1988, Greg Winter developed a special method for humanizing monoclonal antibodies, which made it possible to make molecules from mice more "human-like." Antibodies in which some animal proteins are replaced with human proteins are known as chimeric antibodies. These antibodies are commonly used for therapeutic purposes.

THE NATURAL ANTIGEN CYCLE

Most tumor antigens, for example, the p53 protein, which mutates in cancer cells with particular frequency, "work" inside the cell, in the cytoplasm or in the nucleus. How is it that the immune system manages to recognize them when immune cells, whether macrophages or T-cells, only come into contact with the tumor's surface? The secret of that clairvoyance was only discovered in the late twentieth century and was directly connected to the fundamental property of living matter of its continuous self-renewal. It is not only the organism as a whole that lives based on the timely disposal of deteriorated, aged cells. Each of these cells is also constantly renewing its contents. Some biomolecules exist for just a few minutes, while others exist for hours, but in the end, they are all consumed. Using roughly the same mechanisms that our common ancestors — amoebas — used to digest food, the cells of multicellular organisms are constantly renewing themselves: "old" cells are "digested" and new ones are synthesized.

Disposing of unnecessary macromolecules takes place in several stages. First, the proteins are split into short fragments called peptides. Then, most of the peptides are broken down into amino acids, which are recycled by the resourceful cells. However, some "undigested" peptides will form complexes with special proteins, collectively known as proteins of the "major histocompatibility complex" (MHC), which have a common structural motif — a "gap" that is capable of binding to short peptides.

Once the MHC has bound to peptides, it is sent together with them to the cell surface, where it remains for some time, and then returns to the cytoplasm where it is in turn decomposed into amino acids. Thus, any organism cell continuously represents random fragments on its surface of all the proteins stably synthesized within it in real time, forming a dynamic "peptide portrait" or "peptide catalogue" of its vital activity.

See how beautifully it all works out. The infected (or cancerous) cell does not aspire to display any foreign macromolecule fragments on its surface. In fact, it actually has no idea which of the proteins inside it is not like the others, but simply displays everything it has. Researchers believe that during infection, out of approximately one hundred thousand MHC molecules present on the cell surface, peptides from foreign proteins bound to the complex will make up just one hundred molecules or so. For tumor antigens, this ratio is probably even lower, but even such a negligible sign of "foreignness" is sufficient for T-cells to recognize the enemy and attack it.

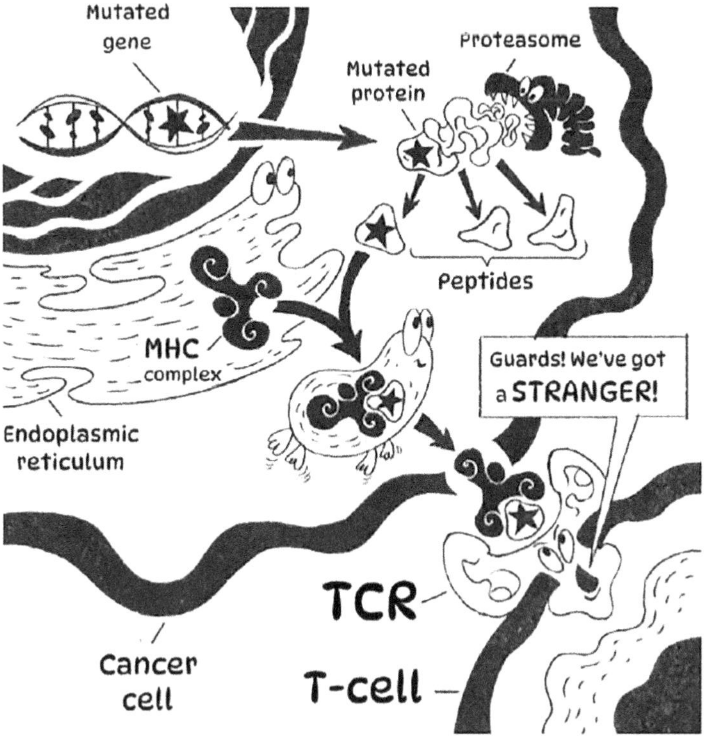

Figure 18. TCRs recognize cancer antigens (fragments of mutated proteins) in the MHC complex. Recognizing foreign proteins (cancerous as well as viral and bacterial) activates the immune response and the immune system destroys the suspicious cell.

FACT: The two types of immunity – innate and acquired – are intertwined. In order to activate lymphocytes, they need the support of dendritic cells and macrophages, while antibodies and cytokines produced by lymphocytes help the innate immune system destroy any enemies.

Allergies are a disease of clean hands

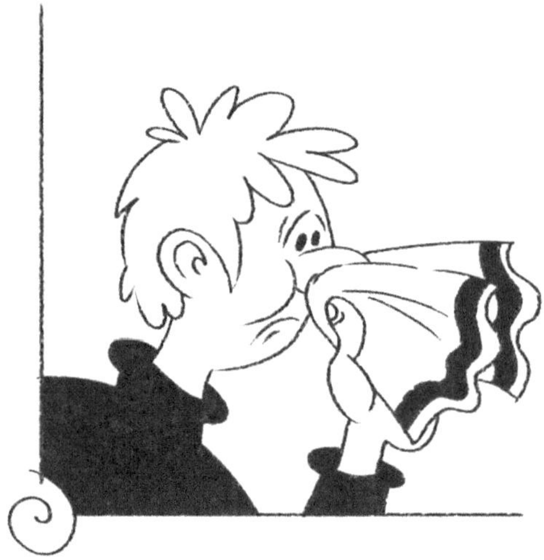

In countries that are capable of providing their citizens with the opportunity to follow hygienic standards and timely access to medical care, many diseases are gradually disappearing. But there is one group of diseases that is being diagnosed with increasing frequency among people in rich, developed countries, and that is allergies of all stripes. Unlike normal immune reactions, which fight real enemies of the body by creating a destructive effect, an allergic reaction is an over-excitement in the presence of perfectly innocent antigens. We are all familiar with plant pollen, which can make patients' lives "extra fun" to the tune of "with friends like these, who needs enemies?"

Household, food, and drug allergies are so widespread today that it is hard for us to imagine that during the early twentieth century they were a rare disease, usually confined to members of high society. The rapid growth of allergies after World War II drove scientists to look for an explanation for the phenomenon. One of the most convincing theories to date is the so-called "hygiene hypothesis," suggested in 1989 by David Strachan. Strachan studied the incidence of allergic rhinitis (hay fever) and concluded that the more children there were in a family, the less likely a child would be to develop the allergy. Strachan believed that this was because children in large families are inevitably exposed to all sorts of infections from their siblings at a young age, which contributes to their immune systems' ability to adequately adjust.

The human body was formed in conditions that were very different from the sterility that has become the standard in developed countries. If, during this sensitive period of early childhood, the immune system is not given the opportunity to interact with the appropriate number of antigens, it acquires hypersensitivity, which later manifests as allergies, much as a spoiled child raised in a golden cage by people who are always ready to cater to their every whim begins to throw a tantrum any time someone does not agree with them. This is why rural children suffer from allergies less often than those raised in the city, people who live in developing countries suffer less than Europeans and North Americans, and immigrants from developing countries who move to wealthier regions begin to suffer more from immune disorders the longer they live in their new environment.

Today, immunologists unanimously advise parents to avoid creating an environment that is too sterile around young children. Digging in the dirt, trying to pet any small animal that might run by, and putting sticks they find on the ground in their mouth are not only a way to explore the world, but also a way to train the immune system. A few dozen childhood infections at a young age, along with lice and worms — the usual companions to socializing in a school environment — are a small price to pay for the freedom to eat what you like, have pets, and enjoy the springtime bloom with delight, rather than tears.

TUMORS AND IMMUNITY – AN EVOLUTIONARY DIALOGUE

If the methods for recognizing any sign of molecular foreignness in the human body are so perfect, why, then, do we still get cancer? Why does our immune system not simply put a spoke in the tumor's wheel? Why is it allowed to grow? There is no one simple answer to that question, though there are several complicated ones.

First of all, the immune system appears to destroy a huge number of microtumors, thereby preventing them from growing and causing problems for the body. Cancer is still the "exception" rather than the "rule" for a healthy body. At the same time, data on people suffering from AIDS and experiments with immunodeficient animals show that a weakened immune system can lead to dramatic growth in tumors, especially those that are viral in nature. One such tumor, Kaposi's sarcoma, is a typical symptom of the transition from a slow-growing and virtually asymptomatic HIV infection to the terminal stage known as full-blown AIDS.

Second, recognizing and eliminating foreign agents, whether infections or malignant tumors, generally follows the same pattern, while the immune response in cancer has its own characteristics. Cancer cells are too similar to normal body cells, and the immune system's reaction to the few tumor antigens will be much less pronounced than in the case of an infection, in which nearly any viral or bacterial protein is a foreign agent triggering an immune response.

Third, as we have already learned, cancer is a disease of the elderly, and as we age, so does the rest of our body, including our immune system. It may be that the increase in cancer cases with age is linked not only to accumulating genetic errors in the body cells, but also a weakened ability to recognize and destroy malignant cells.

Finally, a tumor is not static, but rather a dynamic, developing structure. Cancer cells are highly variable and gradually change the tumor's properties in such a way that it is able to effectively resist the immune response, and, unfortunately, the body's defenses are not always the winners of this "arms race."

In the early twentieth century, renowned scientist Theodosius Dobzhansky stated: "Nothing in biology makes any sense, except in light of evolution." This generalization is not only true for events in the biological "macroworld"—changes in individuals and species — but the same evolutionary laws can also be applied to tumors, when it comes to the cells on which the body's immune system acts (even before chemotherapy has begun) as a factor of Darwinian natural selection. The evolutionary "dialogue" between groups of overgrown cells (a future tumor) and the body develops in several stages. At the beginning, most of the action takes place in the body's defense forces, while at the end (once the disease has developed) it completely moves to the tumor itself. Just a few years ago, researchers described the main stages of this process as part of the concept of the tumor undergoing "immune editing."

The first stage of immune editing is a process of elimination. Under the influence of internal or external factors, normal cells will transform, becoming capable of unlimited division, no longer responding to the body's regulatory signals. At the same time, they generally begin to synthesize "tumor antigens" and "danger signals" on their surface. These signals attract immune system cells, primarily macrophages, the body's natural killers, and T-cells. In most cases, the immune system is able to successfully destroy the "tainted" cells and interrupt the tumor development at a precancerous stage. However, sometimes there are some precancerous cells among them with a weakened ability to trigger an immune response. They synthesize fewer tumor agents, are less likely to be recognized by the immune system, and after surviving the first wave of immune response, they will continue to develop. When this occurs, the interaction between the tumor and body reaches the second stage: equilibrium.

During this stage, the immune system is no longer capable of completely destroying the tumor, but it is still able to limit its growth. In this "equilibrium" (which is undetectable by most diagnostic methods), microtumors can exist in the body for years. However, these latent tumors are not static. The properties of their cells will gradually change under the influence of mutations and subsequent selection, and those that are better capable of resisting the immune system gain an advantage. In the end, immunosuppressor cells will appear in the tumor, able to not only passively avoid destruction, but actively thwart the immune response.

Thus, in its attempt to beat the disease, like a careless mad scientist from a fantasy thriller, the body will accidentally "breed" a super predator capable of resisting any enemy from what began as a rather harmless tumor. (From an evolutionary perspective, the process of "breeding" antibiotic-resistant bacteria by misusing medications looks a lot like this.)

This dramatic moment marks the transition of a malignant neoplasm to the third stage of development — the immune-response-avoidance stage, which is a key sign of cancer. During this stage, the tumor is no longer sensitive to the immune system cells' activities and is in fact capable of using that activity to its advantage. The cancerous tumor begins to grow and spread throughout the body. This is the stage when the tumor is usually diagnosed by doctors and studied by scientists — the previous stages are latent and our understanding of them is mainly based on indirect, experimental data.

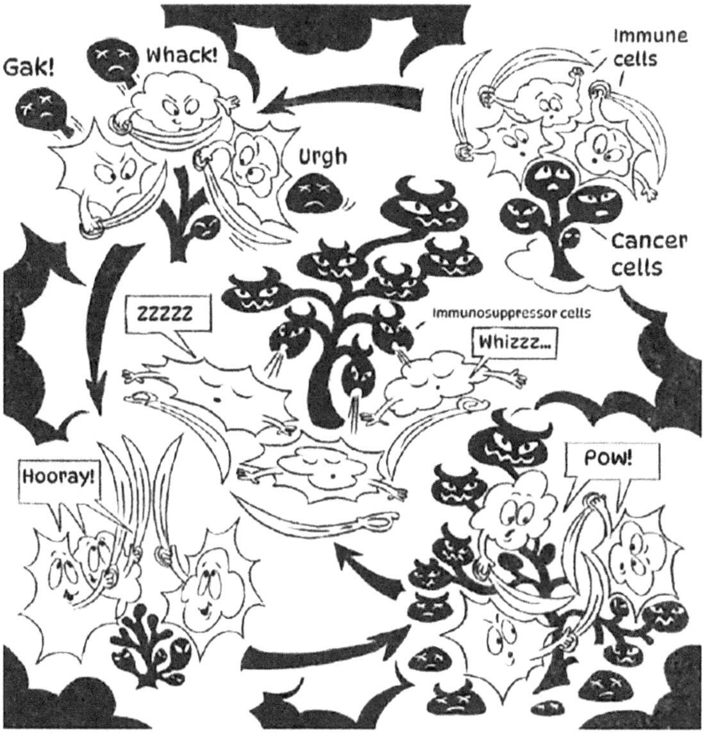

Figure 19. Tumor evolution. Confrontation between cancer cells and the immune response leads to the tumor becoming more effective at resisting attacks from immune cells. During the initial (latent) stage of the disease, leukocytes are able to easily destroy most of the precancerous and cancerous cells and thereby slow down tumor growth. However, during later stages, as a result of natural selection, cells capable of both being "invisible" to the immune system and effectively suppressing the immune response appear in the neoplasm, and the tumor begins to rapidly and uncontrollably grow in size. Avoiding immune control is a key hallmark of cancer (see Figure 1).

Fortunately, research over the last few decades has shown that it is possible to try to resuscitate a suppressed immune response within a tumor. This is the aim of the new generation of anti-cancer immunotherapy drugs.

FACT: As a malignant tumor evolves, its ability to suppress the immune response also changes.

THE IMMUNE RESPONSE FORMULA

Chemists say that "dirt is a substance that is out of place." We need to keep that principle in mind as we think about the behavior of malignant tumors. Based on the description of how cancer evolves, it might seem that cancer cells are extraordinarily ingenious. However, that is decidedly not the case! By nature, the tumor is not ingenious, but a plagiarist.

A depressed immune system in itself is not necessarily a bad thing. On the contrary, though, an out-of-control immune system has incredibly destructive power. The most dangerous infection will usually take several days to kill a person, but the most severe type of allergic reaction — anaphylactic shock — can do that within a few minutes. Timely suppression is a natural part of a normal immune response to avoid unnecessary and excessive destruction of the body. The "secret" to a malignant tumor's success is that it abuses these healthy molecular mechanisms. A classic example of that is the way that macrophages are reprogrammed in the tumor environment.

When we talk about the immune response, we usually use a lot of military-themed metaphors—"fight," "destroy," "attack." But whether we are dealing with a virus, bacteria, or parasite, destroying the enemy is not enough. The body also needs to repair the damage that has been caused. The immune system cells also control regenerating tissue and healing wounds: in our body, it is not only a soldier, but also a healer. The same type of cell — macrophages — can play either of these roles, depending on what the body needs. M1 macrophages (also known as classically activated macrophages) are the "warriors," and responsible for destroying foreign agents (including tumor cells), either directly or by attracting and activating other immune system cells (such as killer T-cells). M2 macrophages are the "healers," which accelerate tissue regeneration and heal wounds.

The presence of a large number of M1 macrophages within a tumor will slow down its growth, and in some cases even cause almost complete remission (elimination). On the contrary, M2 macrophages will produce molecules that stimulate tumor cell division, which favors the development of a malignant neoplasm.

Experimentation has shown that M2 cells (healers) tend to dominate in the tumor environment. Moreover, when they are under the influence of substances released by tumor cells, active M1 macrophages "reprogram" into M2-type cells. They stop synthesizing anti-tumor cytokines such as interleukin-12 or tumor necrosis factor and instead start releasing molecules into the environment that accelerate tumor growth and the creation of blood vessels to provide it with nutrients, such as the tumor growth factor (TGF⊠) we learned about earlier or the vascular endothelial growth factor (VEGF). M2 macrophages stop activating T-cells and other immune system cells, and instead start blocking the local (anti-tumor) immune response. As is the case with other cells in the tumor environment, cancer's insidiousness lies in the fact that it is essentially a "foreign agent," but presents itself to the body in a way that leukocytes believe it is not an enemy to destroy, but an unhealed wound needing help, protection, and healing.

FACT: In some tumors, macrophages make up 50 percent of the cellular content.

BRINGING IMMUNITY BACK TO CANCER

Another example of the molecular "switch" that cancer cells use to serve their own needs are the T-cell membrane proteins known as "immunity checkpoints" (not to be confused with "cell cycle checkpoints"!).

T-cells are the main group of adaptive (acquired) immune cells in vertebrates. Their "combat unit" is made up of cytotoxic T-cells (also known as killer T-cells), which ensure that they recognize and destroy cells carrying foreign antigens on their surface, including tumor cells. However, "naïve" and "untrained" T-cells are not initially able to recognize antigens directly on the tumor's surface. Instead, they must "learn" this with the help of a special group of innate immunity cells known as antigen-presenting cells, which consist of dendritic cells and macrophages. During the primary immune response, they attack the tumor and devour the dead cancer cells. They then begin to display both their own peptides and the peptides of the digested tumor cells, including tumor antigens, on their surfaces (if the person is lucky).

A foreign peptide on the surface of a dendritic cell (or macrophage) within the MHC complex interacts with the TCRs on all available T-cells, until it meets the most suitable one among them, in which the TCR can most efficiently bind to that antigen.

However, the mere presence of a foreign antigen is not enough to fully activate the T-cell response. Much like when we have to sign a loan agreement for a large sum of money at the bank and produce additional ID documents to guarantee we are solvent, the T-cells require "additional confirmation" in the form of special activation molecules, which are also synthesized by dendritic cells and macrophages.

The most well-known T-cell response co-activation molecules are B7 proteins. These membrane proteins bind to CD28 receptors on a T-cell's surface, temporarily "gluing" two cells together. This additional "molecular stitching" is necessary in order to activate the immune response; without it, the T-cell will not activate.

However, as we described earlier, timely suppression of the immune response is a natural part of this system. Nearly immediately after it is activated in the T-cells, processes are triggered to inhibit and limit their protective but also destructive activities. Activated T-cells begin expressing CTLA4 proteins. These are a "close relative" and also a competitor of CD28 receptors. CTLA4 interacts with the same activator molecules (B7) as CD28, but is much more efficient, and as a result B7 proteins' co-activation of the T-cells weakens the immune response and causes it to subside.

As it acts together with antigen-recognition receptor TCR, CD28 activates a range of intracellular kinases (enzymes that phosphorylate other proteins), while the CTLA4 signal leads to the activation of their "molecular antagonists", phosphatases (enzymes that dephosphorylate other proteins). This receptor thus slows down the immune response in the membranes as well as at the intracellular level. This molecular "safeguard" is unusually important for limiting the development of a pathologically strong immune response. Mice in which the CTLA4 gene was artificially turned off died of systemic autoimmune reactions — they literally killed themselves.

Another checkpoint for inhibiting T-cell response is the PD-1 receptor. Just like CTLA4, PD-1 is not expressed on the surface of "naïve" T-cells, and begins to synthesize only after the immune response is activated.

The ligands that use this receptor to trigger inhibition of the T-cell response in tumors are actively produced not only by cancer cells, but also by the other immune cells present, such as macrophages and dendritic cells This is another example of "reprogramming" when cells in the tumor environment which should in theory fight off the malignant transformation instead begin "working for the enemy."

Studying tumors' mechanisms of avoiding the immune system response led scientists to develop drugs that regulate inhibitory checkpoints in T-cells. Researchers suggested that blocking these receptors might potentially restore normal immune cells' activity and strengthen their anti-tumor activity. The first articles about this topic appeared in the late 1990s, but it is a long road between a scientific idea and the release of a new drug. It was not until 2011 that the US Food and Drug Administration approved the release of the first drug of this group, ipilimumab (which blocks CTLA4), and in 2014 it approved the drug nivolumab (which blocks PD-1). We have already discussed both of these drugs, which are monoclonal antibodies to the corresponding proteins. Currently, they have only been approved for the treatment of melanoma, but clinical trials are underway for possibly using them to treat prostate, lung, and kidney cancers. Each of them shows high efficacy for treating metastatic melanoma, and their combined use greatly enhances their pharmaceutical effect.

Scientists are currently looking with great interest at other inhibitory receptors that might be capable of using their blocking mechanism to strengthen the immune system's anti-tumor response. Today, natural killer inhibitor receptors, along with LAG3, TIM3, and CD276 proteins, are seen as promising targets for immunotherapy. Scientists hope that in the next few years, they will have new drugs capable of pinpointing their action to consolidate the success of this type of immunotherapy and give many patients a chance at prolonging their lives.

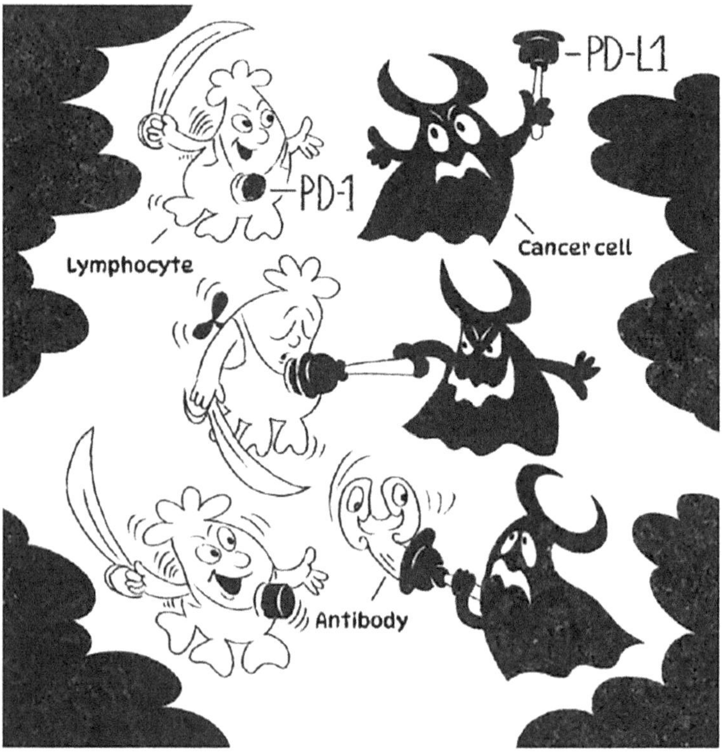

Figure 20. PD-1 protein is present on the surface of T-cells, and PD-L1 protein is present on the surface of cancer cells. When these proteins interact, the lymphocyte is "turned off" and the T-cell stops attacking. Normally, this molecular mechanism of immune response inhibition is necessary in order to keep active lymphocytes under control and ensure they do not destroy the organism. But cancer cells take advantage of them to serve their own purposes. Therapeutic antibodies ("immune response checkpoint inhibitors") stick to PD-L1 proteins and prevent them from interacting with PD-1. This is how T-cells remain active and are capable of effectively destroying the tumor cells.

One alternative method for activating the adaptive immune system in a tumor is using chimeric antigen receptor (CAR) technology, in which artificial chimeric proteins capable of effectively recognizing tumor antigens are "sewn" onto the patient's own T-cells. This treatment has already been approved for treating several types of malignant blood diseases and shown itself to be highly effective for late-stage leukemia and lymphoma. This treatment is an extremely expensive (as the cells are constructed individually for each patient) but very promising immunotherapy method.

The 2018 Nobel Prize in Physiology or Medicine was shared by American immunologist James Allison, who researched the properties of CTLA4, and Japanese immunologist Tasuku Honjo, who discovered the PD-1 protein. Many scientists believe that the authors of CAR technology also have a shot at winning this prestigious scientific award in the coming years.

FACT: The two most modern methods for activating anti-cancer immunity are therapies based on controlling immune checkpoints and CAR technology. So far, however, they have shown to be effective in treating only a few types of cancer.

WHY CANCER IMMUNOTHERAPY IS NOT INVINCIBLE (YET...?)

As we pay tribute to the successes of modern immunotherapy, we cannot lose sight of the fact that it is still very early to talk about it as a universal treatment method. The key problem lies in the fact that the immune system can only be strengthened if it exists in principle. And for that, the tumor must first synthesize enough antigens, and then these antigens must be present on the cell surface.

However, not all tumors synthesize tumor antigens. In some cancers, mutations only affect the regulatory regions of DNA and the transformation is not linked with changes to the protein structure, but only disruptions to their regulation. Other tumors simply hide their antigens.

From the perspective of the malignant neoplasm's interests, no tumor antigen on the cell surface — no problem! There are several ways for the cancer cell to achieve this result. It might disrupt the cellular protein digestion process. It might damage protein transporters responsible for delivering peptides from the cytosol, where proteins are digested into the endoplasmic reticulum, where, in turn, MHC complexes gather. Finally, it can disrupt the expression of MHC proteins themselves. All of these pathways lead to one result — the process of normal presentation of peptides (including tumor antigens) on the surface of these cells is disrupted. As long as T-cells are not able to recognize antigens other than as part of the MHC complex, those tumor cells and their antigens will become "invisible" to the T-cell response, and as a result, they will lose sensitivity to immunotherapy. Today, immunology faces the question if these "invisible" tumors can be made "visible" to the immune system once again? Many lives will be saved if they can.

FACT: The term "antigen" was suggested in the early twentieth century by Hungarian microbiologist László Detre in an article coauthored with renowned Russian scientist Ilya Mechnikov.

CANCER IS CONTAGIOUS BUT NOT IN HUMANS!

The most impressive examples of how cancer is capable of cheating the immune system are seen in the transmissible or "contagious" cancers that exist in nature. Tumors are malignant neoplasms that can be transmitted from one organism to another. Fortunately, that almost never happens in humans. In the early days of organ transplants, there were cases described where a person received an organ with metastasis lurking, which led to the development of cancer. But that kind of infection is only possible in the context of the powerful immunosuppressive therapy that transplant patients undergo in order to prevent organ rejection. Today, transplant surgeons avoid using organs from people who have had cancer, which reduces the risk of infection to almost zero. There are no other types of "contagious cancers" in humans.

Other species are much less fortunate. An epidemic of what scientists describe as "contagious cancer" drove one species of marsupial, the Tasmanian devil, to the brink of extinction. The disease, known as "devil facial tumor disease," was described in Australia in the late 1990s. The disease first affects the skin on the animal's face and mucous membranes of the mouth, before growing rapidly and metastasizing to the internal organs, mostly the lungs. This is an absolutely lethal disease, and within a few months after infection, the Tasmanian devil dies of starvation, suffocation, or malignant tumors in the internal organs.

Over the last few decades, the epidemic has reduced the already-small population of these animals to critical levels in some places. The tumor's rapid spread is related to the Tasmanian devils' behavior — they often bite one another when mating or eating together, and easily spread tumor cells from the mouth of a sick animal into a wound in the mouth of a healthy one. Today, ecologists are trying to save the species from extinction by isolating a small population of completely healthy animals and creating favorable conditions for them to reproduce. At the same time, immunologists are trying to understand why the cells of these tumors are not rejected when they make it into another animal, as usually happens in organ or tissue transplants.

Initially, it was thought that high rates of inbreeding among Tasmanian devils played an important role in spreading the disease, as all of the animals would have a high level of shared genetic identity as close relatives. But it is now clear that this cannot explain everything. After all, if one tries to transplant a piece of healthy skin from one Tasmanian devil to another, it will be rejected, though for some reason this does not happen with cancer.

Another example of contagious cancer is canine transmissible venereal tumors, which, as the name implies, are transmitted from one animal to another when mating. Unlike the scourge decimating the Tasmanian devils, which emerged fairly recently, dogs have suffered from this disease for thousands of years.

Fortunately, this tumor does not threaten our four-legged friends in the same numbers and is not as aggressive as the Tasmanian devils' tumor. It is also treatable, though in terms of "classical immunology," its appearance and spread look just as inexplicable.

Scientists believe that studying these "exotic" diseases will help them better understand the molecular mechanisms of common (non-contagious) tumors escaping immune control and think of new ways we can prevent that from happening.

FACT: Some very rare cancers are contagious; that is, they can be transmitted from one individual to another within the same species. Fortunately, this does not happen in humans.

SUMMARY

In this chapter, we learned about the features of the immune response in cancer and some of the molecular mechanisms that tumors use in order to evade that response. We got to know some of the main methods for stimulating the immune system against tumors. Generally speaking, our conversation about the "warped mirror of life" can be considered complete. However, before we finish our journey through the world of molecular oncology, we need to address the popular myth stating that scientists already know everything, but they are just hiding it all. We will conclude this book with a brief explanation of how modern science works and why it is impossible to have any secret knowledge that is inaccessible to those who are uninitiated.

Chapter 8. A BRAVE NEW WORLD AND CONSPIRACY THEORIES IN ONCOLOGY

Whether or not they actually explain cancer or the universe, "alternative theories" cannot exist without attacking the scientific worldview. In the case of cancer, those attacks tend to masquerade as criticism of the current healthcare system and pharmaceutical industry in general.

Many of those criticisms are fair; pharmaceutical companies are indeed sometimes more worried about profits than saving human lives. For this reason, they only very rarely invest in developing medicines for rare diseases, as the cost of research for a high-demand drug will be the same, with much greater returns, given the large number of patients. And there is hardly a single country on earth where citizens are entirely satisfied with the quality of their healthcare system. However, the myth makers out there take advantage of people's natural tendency to be dissatisfied with the existing order of things to spread ideas that have nothing to do with reality. These myths are no different from political conspiracies about secretive cabals with evil designs on the rest of humanity, and could be described as myths about a global conspiracy in Western medicine and pharmaceutical companies. The main idea behind this myth is that a universal cancer cure already exists (or is about to be invented), but corrupt medical professionals and greedy pharmaceutical companies are hiding it from us all. A milder version of this myth might sound something like: "Alternative methods (like the baking soda idea we discussed earlier) are much more effective than the treatments accepted by Western medicine, but corrupt medical professionals and greedy pharmaceutical companies..."

In order to understand why these claims cannot possibly be true, we will look at the principles of evidence-based medicine, learn about modern methods for drug development, and realize that, sooner or later, someone will let the cat out of the bag, and that the main trend in modern oncology is not creating a one-size-fits-all magic pill to cure all types of cancer, but the development of specific, targeted drugs based on what we know about the molecular features of each patient's disease. In the future, this "personalized" or "precision" approach to medicine will probably expand to include other complicated and multifactor diseases. A brief overview of the latest medical technology based on big data will conclude our journey into the world of molecular oncology.

WHAT EVIDENCE IS THERE TO EVIDENCE-BASED MEDICINE?

Post hoc, ergo propter hoc. This Latin expression means "after this, therefore because of this," or rather, if y follows x, x must have caused y. This is one of the most common fallacies that people encounter every day. Writer Nassim Taleb draws a connection to our mind's need to build a "narrative," or the desire to describe the chaos of reality within some sort of structure — to tell a "story" dictated by causal connections (most of them fictional).

"I took XXX and that is what cured me." This is the most common way we see drug effectiveness reviewed, but what is wrong with this statement? Apart from the survivor error we described earlier (have most of the people who took XXX recovered or is the narrator the only one to be so lucky?), it points to a causal link that may not exist. As they say, "If you treat a runny nose, it will go away in seven days, but if you let it run its course, you'll be better in a week." Spontaneous remission does not only happen with cancer. Moreover, while with cancer it is about as likely as a miracle, the same phenomenon is in fact quite common in many other, less serious conditions. Finally, it is possible that the narrator was already on the road to recovery, and the XXX they took had nothing to do with it at all.

Beyond any miracle cure, there might be other important factors that are actually improving someone's health. For example, in acute respiratory infections, whether or not a patient is drinking enough fluids is a major factor that will have a great impact on alleviating their symptoms. A patient who took a placebo and also drank a lot of water might really feel better, but it is not due to the "medication" (which did not have any effective ingredients, anyway), but the fluids, which were not given any credit. Finally, humans are social animals, with highly complex mental processes that have a significant effect on our physical well-being. A placebo effect occurs when a patient feels better, simply because they know they are being treated, despite the fact that the drugs they are taking have no active ingredients. After having a conversation with a sympathetic doctor willing to lend them an ear, many elder retirees who have been suffering from social isolation suddenly feel better. "Kind words heal and help"—people have known this since the beginning of time. But we should be able to discern the "kind words" effect from an actual, medicinal effect, which will work regardless of a doctor's bedside manner.

All of the above should make it clear that a single (however successful!) experience with a drug is in no way enough to prove whether or not it is effective. In order to prove that the drug actually works, we must conduct a study on a group of patients large enough to ensure that the trial results are statistically significant. These experiments are known as clinical trials.

The gold standard for testing drug effectiveness is an approach known as a double-blind placebo-controlled trial. The word "blind" here means that the patients taking part in the trial do not know if they are getting the actual drug being tested or a sham, or placebo. "Double-blind" implies that the healthcare professionals working on the study also do not know which drug the patients are getting. All names of the drug samples are encrypted and can only be deciphered after the trial has been completed, when data on the treatment's effectiveness has already been gathered. This approach minimizes the interference of personal factors on the part of the patients or physicians and means that the clinical experiment will be as close to a laboratory experiment as possible. When testing a new drug for a disease for which there is already an approved treatment, the known drug will be used rather than a placebo and compared to the new drug being studied. Is it more effective? Safer?

Drugs that do not pass such rigorous testing are by default considered drugs with unproven clinical benefits, and ideally should not be prescribed by doctors.

In the real world, not everyone has access to high-quality medical care, and it is often a situation of the blind leading the blind. It is useful to keep in mind that there are international treatment protocols for certain diseases (including cancer), based on the medical community's global experience (and the results of clinical trials). Information on these international standards is available online, on the Guidelines International Network, a global databank of treatment and diagnostic recommendations and guidelines.

Information is also open and available on clinical trials underway around the world. The American Cancer Society provides information on clinical trials for cancer treatments in which interested patients with the right diagnoses can participate.

The use of statistical methods to objectively analyze drug efficacy is just the tip of the iceberg, and the mark of modern biology's shift toward rigor and precision. This is how biology tries to respond to current challenges, the most serious of which is the issue of big data.

FACT: All homeopathic medicine is medicine with unproven efficacy.

A QUIET REVOLUTION — BIG DATA IN MOLECULAR ONCOLOGY

We are living in an era of revolution, but it is a quiet, creeping social shift that only rarely shows up in public scandals like the debate over social media's influence on the 2016 US presidential elections. The old political players still retain their influence, but those who own data and know how to use it hold a new and by no means illusive power, which will only grow with time. Big data is changing the rules of the political game and influencing the economy as well as our social lives. When it comes to science, the use of big data in biology has led to radical changes right before the eyes of just one generation of scientists.

Just twenty or thirty years ago, to say nothing of even further back in history (an insignificant period by historical standards), the main problem of molecular biology was the acute lack of experimental results. Purifying and crystallizing proteins and obtaining information about their spatial structure was a difficult mystery that took a long time to crack, much like alchemical transformation. Sequencing (decoding the sequence) of genes or proteins was a multi-month project worthy of its own article. Theoretical biology was developing predictive algorithms for anything and everything. Predictions, however imprecise, were in high demand, as they at least made it possible to cover and patch up some of the gaping holes in what we knew.

The advent of new methods eventually improved science's productivity, but this was a slow, gradual process. The first protein crystallization was awarded the Nobel Prize, but just a few decades later (again — decades!), this task has become a rather mundane thesis topic in just about any highly ranked university. Scientific data was accumulated and thought about for a long time. There was a time, and there are plenty of witnesses who are still alive, when it was considered to be a good idea for any scientist studying protein spatial structure patterns to memorize (in general) the structures of all known proteins. Today, that would simply be impossible to imagine.

The information we have about the dynamic properties of living systems has also accumulated slowly. What will a certain protein interact with? How does any given gene's activity change during biological processes? Answering each required a series of complicated experiments.

All of that dramatically changed very quickly. Experimental methods appeared which made it possible to analyze the expression of tens of thousands of genes at the same time, track the behavior of thousands of proteins, and monitor mutations in the entire genome. The results from these highly productive experiments expanded what we know about the molecular foundations of life, while simultaneously becoming a source of a rather new systemic crisis that modern thinkers consider as "self-shadowing of science."

Sometimes, as we scroll through pages and pages of articles generated by a small query on a search engine, we cannot help but wonder — perhaps we already have all we need to understand life, but the information is simply poorly organized... Molecular biology no longer suffered from a data deficit. It began to choke on all the data available, crushed by the excess of it. Molecular oncology was not spared from this crisis.

What could we learn about a particular tumor using the methods of "classical" molecular biology? We could check the typical mutations — p53, BRCA, etc. We could look at the expression level of certain ligands and growth factor and hormone receptors in order to understand exactly which signal pathways were accelerating cellular division; determine the metabolism features; check the markers of immune cell presence; and draw conclusions about the patient's immune status. We have already discussed all of these methods, and many of them are now part of everyday clinical practices.

What capabilities does cutting-edge biology give us to characterize a single tumor? First of all, we can sequence the entire tumor genome and check for mutations in ALL of the genes (not only in known oncogenes and oncosuppressors). Second, we can measure the activity level in ALL of the tumor genes, once again, and look at how they changed, for example, in response to treatment. When we say ALL of the genes, this is about twenty thousand. We get twenty thousand sets of data from the study of a single tumor (and probably more), rather than just twenty to thirty (and that is if you get the maximum) parameters through classical methods. Are you starting to see the scale of the problem?

And this is just a preview. In recent years, technology for a "cell-by-cell" analysis has developed rapidly, making it possible to study the level of gene activity not in the sample as a whole, but in each specific cell. Using this method on one tissue sample, it is possible to collect not twenty thousand sets of data, but twenty thousand multiplied by N, where N is the number of cells, and not necessarily even just cancer cells. This method can also be used in order to characterize the quality of the cellular microenvironment. But once again, we are still talking about just one patient and one tumor sample — and there are potentially millions of patients and tumors around the world, just like this, and sometimes they have more than just one tumor...

This is how huge tables full of endless rows of data are born. There are seas and entire oceans of information, but modern biology does not feel so much like a fish in the water as someone who is drowning and trying to reach the shore. Information is not the same as knowledge — far from it! In order to transform the former into the latter, we need to dedicate an enormous amount of intellectual effort, and the results are by no means guaranteed. Today, there is a huge gap between the immense power of high-performance methods and the limited capabilities of existing approaches to explain and use all of the data they crank out.

Right now, in hundreds and thousands of laboratories around the world, experts are combining biological knowledge with the mastery of advanced information technology — bioinformatics — looking at how to get these new mountains of data to “speak.” There is no doubt that biology in the twenty-first century will be a big data science. Molecular oncology is a testing ground for advanced methods that will later expand to include other areas of life science.

FACT: Global job market trends suggest that bioinformatics and data analysis experts will be among the most in-demand professionals in the near future.

IN BOTH NUMBERS AND SKILL!

Of course, there is no point in thinking about new technologies as some kind of disaster. It is true that the advent of high-performance methods has led to some bottlenecks in basic science, but the success of their applications has exceeded anyone's wildest expectations. New technologies radically accelerated the development of drugs, including for cancer treatment.

For centuries, seeking potential medicinal substances was a matter of intuition and luck rather than calculation — just look at the history of penicillin, which bacteriologist Alexander Fleming isolated from a mold that grew on a Petri dish containing a bacterial culture; or mustard gas, which led to the advent of chemotherapy. Luck is still a significant factor of success, but today the search for potential drugs has become much more focused. Understanding that at the heart of any physiological process there is a network of certain molecular interactions is what led to the creation of the concept of "drug targets," which is what scientists developing new drugs today are hoping to reach. Drug targets can be more or less accessible by direct action, depending on whether they are on the cell surface, circulating in the blood (like most toxins), or inside the cell. In the first and second case, pharmaceutical research is mostly aimed at searching for and optimizing specific antibodies to this target molecule. Monoclonal antibodies, which we learned about in the previous chapter, take on many pharmaceutical challenges, but not all of them. Searching for drugs that will act on targets inside the cell, where proteins cannot penetrate, remains a serious challenge. This is where chemists can lend biologists a hand.

Until the mid-1980s, the biological activity of new drug candidates was usually studied in animals or cell cultures. These studies lasted a long time, and were very limited in terms of number and variety of substances being tested. (During a week of intensive work using this approach, about twenty to fifty compounds could be studied.) Things radically changed with the advent of high-performance screening, which meant that within just a few days it was possible to test hundreds of thousands and even millions of compounds for a specific target. The process of searching for new active molecules became much faster. Generally speaking, screening large, diverse arrays (libraries) of chemicals is one of the first steps of pharmaceutical research. Today, most major pharmaceutical companies and research centers have such collections of substances, and regularly update them with new compounds in order to ensure the most diverse molecular library possible.

Initial screening never gives you a ready-made medication. However, the data obtained on the activity of a specific substance or groups of substances (hits) is a springboard for further searching and optimizing active molecules. Hit optimization often includes synthesizing hundreds and thousands of various compounds, until scientists achieve the desired activity. In order to reduce the number of lab experiments, they use computer-assisted research methods. The analysis of three-dimensional protein structures taken from the Protein Data Bank can often suggest potential points (sites) for binding for future drugs, while additional computer modeling of molecular interactions can predict ways to optimize the design of a substance (or, often, a group of substances) that is capable of binding to those proteins in specific places (known as the biomechanical puzzle), etc.

We would be remiss to ignore the area of drug development based on the sequential "amplification" of active fragment-based drug discovery (FBDD). FBDD tests relatively small molecules, which can be detected using modern biophysical methods despite their weak binding to the target. Further optimization of the fragment includes building up new parts of the future drug in the right direction, which can sometimes turn out to be a much easier task than other approaches. FBDD is a young field of pharmacology, which has made great strides over the last fifteen years, and there are already two cancer treatment drugs available on the market today that were created through these methods — vemurafenib and venetoclax — while at least two dozen molecules that resulted from this type of fragment assembly are currently in clinical trials.

New drug production technologies are increasing the number of pharmaceuticals available and giving doctors a wider range of options to select the best medications to meet each patient's needs.

However, this accelerated development also comes at a price. Doctors today (especially oncologists) do not have the luxury of spending years treating patients with the same old-fashioned methods they learned in medical school. They need to study for their entire lives, to be up to date on the latest developments in medicine in order to best help their patients.

FACT: On average, of five to ten thousand candidate substances taken into development by pharmaceutical companies, only two hundred and fifty will be selected for preclinical trials (animal testing). Of those, only five will be selected for clinical trials, and only one of those will end up a drug for widespread clinical use.

A doctor in your smartphone

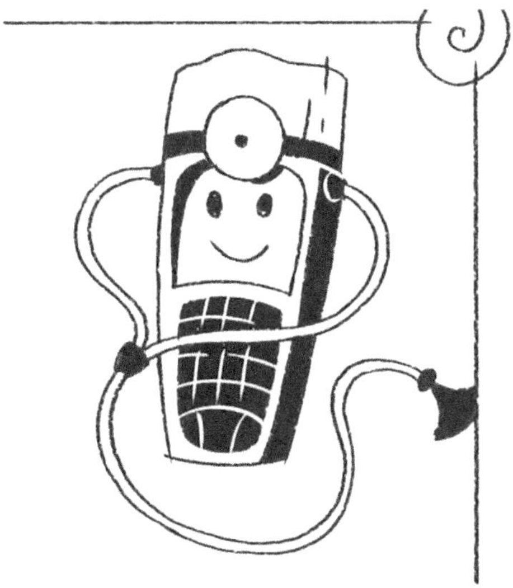

Electronic gadgets and apps today help us stay in touch with the world, but they also help us organize our personal lives, monitor how many calories we consume, and recommend how to maintain optimum physical activity levels. It will not be long before they are used as pocket medical consultants, capable of signaling that a problem has begun before it becomes apparent. (Early diagnosis is the key to successfully treating most diseases, not just cancer.)

In recent years, mobile phone app stores have begun to sell programs that make it possible to early diagnose Parkinson's disease, a severe neurological disorder associated with disruptions to the production of the neurotransmitter dopamine. Late-stage symptoms include a pronounced hand tremor (the original name for Parkinson's was "shaking palsy"). However, before that stage, there is a period of latent development, during which the patient experiences problems with fine motor skills, though the first symptoms are usually not noticeable to the patient. Using a mobile phone — dialing a number, sending a text message — involves many fine, precise movements. By collecting statistics about the user's normal motor activity, the app can "sound the alarm" by detecting that their movements have become less precise or slower, at a stage when the patient is not usually aware of the impairment, yet.

Similar apps are also in development to monitor cancer patients' conditions: following surgery and successful chemotherapy, they are asked to perform a self-diagnosis each day using some simple parameters — if they feel any pain, changes in their weight, mood, etc., in order to not miss any possible return of the disease. Of course, these apps cannot replace face-to-face consultations with a specialist and laboratory diagnostics, but that is not their goal. Their purpose is to improve the quality of care during treatment, which can last for years.

There is also discussion of developing an app to pre-diagnose moles that are suspicious and may become melanomas. By the time this book is published, there will probably already be something available for this. Technology is developing so rapidly that it is impossible for a writer to keep up with it all — God knows that grasping the obvious trends is hard enough! In the coming years, medical app development will make diagnostics more accessible for other diseases. However, their use will only be effective if there is a radical change in attitudes and people get used to the way that new technologies increase our opportunities but also make us take on more responsibility for our own health.

THE CAT'S OUT OF THE BAG

The time has come to address the myth of a global conspiracy in oncopharmacology. Of course, I hope that by now any reader who has reached the final part of this book has already realized that there are many types and causes of cancer, which simply precludes the existence of any single magical cancer cure. Even immunotherapy, which, by definition, is the most universal approach to cancer treatment, includes several different methods and drugs. But just in case, here are a few more arguments that can be used if you ever run into conspiracy theorists (though there is no guarantee that they will see the light).

In order to first address the myth that there is a cure for cancer, but scientists and/or pharmaceutical companies are hiding it from society, common sense and logic are enough. Ordinary people are not the only ones who die of cancer — very rich, famous, and influential people such as Steve Jobs and Patrick Swayze have died from cancer, too. It is hard to imagine that among the developers of a secret super drug, if there really were one, not a single one of them was a fan of Apple or *Dirty Dancing*. It is just as impossible to imagine a pharmaceutical company sitting on that kind of secret and refraining from the temptation to cure such a rich, powerful patient. (A single cure can always be attributed to spontaneous remission, so the risk of being exposed would be negligible, but the potential benefits would be simply enormous.) And yet, to everyone's deep regret, both Jobs and Swayze died.

Any conspiracy theory in science is based on archetypal stories about lone scientists revolutionizing the way we view science. In their day, Pasteur and Fleming certainly could have kept their discoveries secret, which would probably have delayed the advent of rabies vaccines and antibiotics for several decades. But modern science is simply a different animal than it was even a hundred years ago, and even such a specific task as the development of a new drug requires the participation of dozens, if not hundreds, of people, all of them dedicated to seeing their work actually bear fruit. Even if we assume that all of them are die-hard maniacal misanthropes, only concerned with benefiting the pharmaceutical company that hired them — even if we follow Hollywood logic in movies about supervillains — this is simply too far-fetched. A couple of supervillains might be possible, but hundreds is just too much. Of course, a true conspiracy theorist is not going to be convinced by any logical arguments, but fortunately not all of them are quite so stubborn. Let us hope that if you must run into them, they are of the former variety.

Jokes aside, however, there are deeper and much less mundane explanations — rooted in the principles that guide scientific research today — for why modern oncopharmacology (and, more broadly, modern science in general) might sometimes exaggerate its achievements but is incapable of hiding them.

This is not about researchers having any special personal qualities. Basic science is by no means about saints, but is simply full of ordinary people with their own weaknesses and shortcomings. Most research by pharmaceutical companies is focused exclusively on future profits. In both science and the pharmaceuticals industry, there are occasional scandals over fraud (less often than in other fields, but they do happen). But if you look closely at these revelations, it is easy to see that they are almost always related to exaggerations of a certain effect, and never with any understatements. This is no accident.

Let us consider, generally speaking, the process of developing drugs based on active ingredients proposed by chemists. We talked about the technology involved in producing those ingredients earlier. Often, it begins with an independent biological or medical lab. It is rare for pharmaceutical corporations to carry out their own research from scratch; usually, they simply cherry-pick from the results of basic science, and take over from there. Once they have obtained from their colleagues the substances that will bind to the drug target in question, biologists will begin studying their biological activity, first in cell cultures, and later in lab animals — mice or rats.

It is mandatory for scientists to publish the results of their experiments in scientific journals — the number and ranking of scientific articles is the major criterion for success in today's scientific world. What is more, there are so many scientists working in the field of cancer research that, in this field, it is particularly important not only to make a discovery, but to be the first to publish it. Whoever succeeds at that will receive all the glory and grant money for new research. Everyone else will go to another research institute. In these kinds of situations, it would be incredibly costly to hold back any promising results.

If we consider the scientific method, a negative result is still a result, but in practice things are not quite so cheery. Publishing an article full of "not," "does not work," and "does not change," is not very much fun, to say the least. As a result, scientists will try to reinvent the wheel, time and again. Because the results of unsuccessful experiments are almost never published, these tests will have to be repeated, over and over. However, there is a silver lining to all of this wastefulness. On one hand, it is very difficult to publish false reports on the ineffectiveness of a potentially interesting substance, in order to shut things down. Second, if a laboratory is negligent and misses an effect, it will be noticed by another when the experiment is repeated.

If a scientific institute sees any commercial potential in the results of its employees' research, it can patent a specific molecule or method. But patenting is an official and public procedure. In order to protect one's intellectual property, everything has to be made public. If you simply hide all of your discoveries under lock and key, it is highly likely someone else will stumble upon the same discovery. This system (which many researchers are unhappy with) in fact encourages individual scientists who are less than scrupulous to exaggerate their achievements, rather than hide them.

Before an active molecule can become a drug, it must undergo rigorous testing — for toxicity, digestibility, carcinogenicity — and demonstrate that it is effective, first in animal experiments, and later in clinical trials on humans. These tests require a huge financial investment, which can reach several billion dollars. No single laboratory can afford that kind of expense. What is more — biology institutes working with cell cultures and laboratory animals simply do not have the authority to organize clinical trials with patients. This is why after conducting animal experiments and deciding that the method shows good potential, scientists usually offer their developments to a pharmaceutical company.

The pharmaceutical company will study the research results (looking for the quality and number of publications, among other things), and if it looks promising, the company will invest in developing the drug. Is anything being hidden here? Not at all.

Like any business, a pharmaceutical corporation wants to increase its capitalization and attract more market funds. Discovering a new product increases the company's stock value, which is why this information is sure to be advertised with flashing lights in every direction. However, if the candidate drug does not fulfill expectations, that information is likely to be kept quiet until the last possible moment in order to avoid a collapse. Just as in science, the pharmaceutical industry sometimes finds it advantageous to exaggerate successes, never understate them.

There are many large pharmaceutical companies on the market. If they find out that their competitors have begun researching a promising field, the other players will begin their own research in that field. Is the molecule or antibody patented? That is all right — you can always try to find an analogue for the chemical substance or simply synthesize another, similar antibody. Competition and the high cost of running clinical trials keep leading companies from getting too complacent and resting on their laurels. We can look at the example of the current situation of next-generation immunotherapies based on immune response checkpoint inhibitors. In 2011, the company BMS launched its drug ipilimumab (brand name Yervoy), which we have already discussed, on the US market. In 2014, the same company began selling nivolumab (Opdivo). The same year, Merck launched pembrolizumab (Keytruda). In 2016, the Roche corporation, along with Genentech, presented atezolizumab (Tecentriq), and in 2017 two more drugs, avelumab (Bavencio) and durvalumab (Imfinzi) appeared. The first development was the result of cooperation between three major pharmaceutical companies — Merck KGaA, Pfizer, and Eli Lilly. The second was the fruit of cooperation between MedImmune and AstraZeneca. This brief overview of pharmaceutical market news is of course as suspenseful as a report from a marathon: "Runner number 43 is now in the lead... Oh wait, no, now runner 112 has overtaken..." Companies in this "race" are breathing down one another's necks. The winner might not take it all, but they will certainly take a lot. Latecomers will spend billions of dollars in vain — it is much easier to capture an empty market than to try and take a piece of what your competitors have already secured for themselves.

Pharmaceutical corporations will do anything to speed up the release of their drugs on the market. Often, this means that we lose out on detailed research on side effects, and sometimes the drug's effectiveness is exaggerated in unscrupulous advertising. This is not good, but it makes sense from a profit standpoint. But shutting down a drug that is already ready for mass production would surely lead to million-dollar losses and more than a few heads would roll. Companies take such drastic measures only in extreme cases, and never out of concern that the drug "may work too well and then no one would need our other medications." When it does happen, it is always because side effects with the potential for huge lawsuits have surfaced. It is important to keep in mind that it is impossible to evaluate a drug's effectiveness in advance. A drug that has shown itself to be impressively effective in rats might turn out to be quite ineffective in humans. At this stage, the pharmaceutical company simply has nothing to hide, and after clinical trials, it is almost impossible to hide the results. The format of modern medical experiments on humans requires absolute transparency and informed consent from patients and doctors (otherwise the results will simply not be recognized by any official authorities, and all of the money invested will be wasted). The number of people involved in the process at this stage is already in the hundreds, and sometimes in the thousands. What kind of absolute secrecy could we possibly expect here?

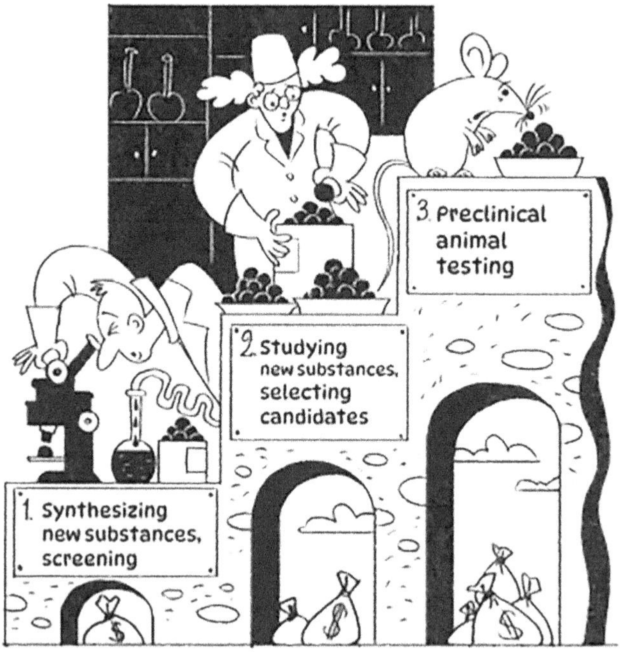

Figure 21. Drug development begins with laboratory experiments and animal testing. Each successive stage of research is several times more expensive than the last one.

This is how the alliance between basic science and applied pharmacology works today. Of course, the disadvantages of this system are visible to the naked eye. The cost of clinical trials is high for new cancer drugs, while the desire to publish at any cost leads to what scientists themselves describe as the "low reproducibility" of many published scientific results. However, one thing is certain — this system eliminates the possibility of any major scientific information (at least, in competitive fields such as molecular oncology) from being concealed. The cat will always find its way out of the bag.

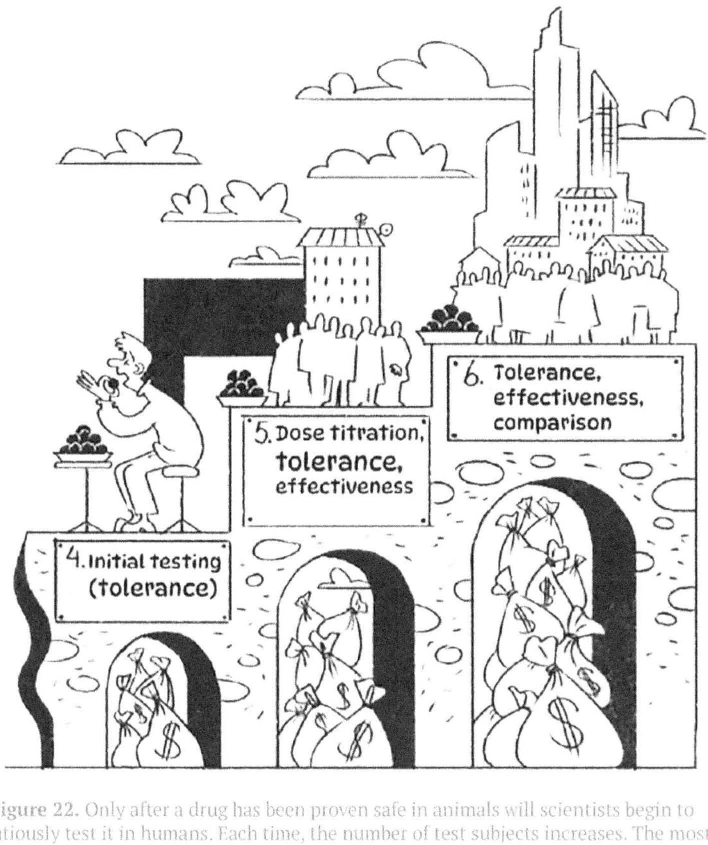

4. Initial testing (tolerance)
5. Dose titration, tolerance, effectiveness
6. Tolerance, effectiveness, comparison

Figure 22. Only after a drug has been proven safe in animals will scientists begin to cautiously test it in humans. Each time, the number of test subjects increases. The most expensive stage of drug development is the large-scale double-blind clinical trial. Once the trial is successful (and not before!), the drug can be approved for sale on the market.

FACT: The most famous case of an already-approved drug being pulled off the market is the story of thalidomide. Thalidomide was a sedative that was perfectly safe in lab animals, but was later found to have teratogenic effects. Women who took the drug during pregnancy gave birth to babies with a range of disabilities, for example, being born with no arms. This resulted in ten thousand children around the world being born with birth defects between 1956 and 1962, forcing many countries to rethink their approach to licensing medications and to tighten their requirements for drug clinical trials. The pharmaceutical company was forced to pay out substantial compensation to the families of the children affected by thalidomide, but those children (who are now adults) continue to file lawsuits against the company.

PRECISION MEDICINE – A BRIGHT FUTURE AWAITS

The rate at which scientific data is growing is changing more than just the face of academic science. Gradually, we are starting to make out the contours of a new approach to treating cancer and other complex diseases at the crossroads of research laboratories, pharmaceutical companies, and medical institutes. That new approach is sometimes known as "precision medicine." The underlying idea is to treat the patient, not the disease.

According to that maxim, by zeroing in on the organism's features due to its unique genotype and personal history, any disease, but especially those as multifactorial and diverse as cancer, acquires individual features that must be addressed if any treatment is going to be successful.

This line of medical thought is not new. The ability to distinguish individual features of any specific disease has always been the skill that separated good and outstanding physicians. However, until recently, there were no methods for objectively qualifying the personal origin factor, or if there were, they were too expensive and difficult to be introduced into mainstream medicine. The advent of powerful high-performance methods, which are growing increasingly affordable, along with just-as-powerful computing systems radically changed the landscape of medical treatment.

Ideally (though this is already foreseeable, and some of it has already even come true), future treatment of cancerous tumors would look like the following: The patient goes to the doctor, who takes a small fragment of the tumor for analysis to determine the tumor's genotype and compare it to the genotype of the patient's healthy cells. Key and associated mutations are identified. At the same time, cells in the tumor's microenvironment are analyzed in order to understand the mechanisms involved in inhibiting the local immune response. Features of local metabolism and blood supply are studied. The results of all these measurements are entered into a special computer program, which analyzes the data based on the information provided on the tumor's sensitivity to various types of drugs, depending on the mutations, type of metabolism, and patient gender and genotype. It then suggests several drug therapy regimens that are capable of mutually reinforcing each other to destroy the tumor and ensure the best immunotherapy option.

The first steps in this direction are already being taken — clinical practice already uses information on frequently mutating genes. Gradually, more and more powerful information technologies are being introduced into medicine, and statistical data on the interaction between various anti-tumor drugs is being gathered and systematized. Information on tumor genotypes, patients, and the effectiveness of various treatments is being gathered into databases and guiding the search for hidden patterns that allow us to enhance the effect of existing drugs.

The main stumbling block right now is the still-exorbitant price of these new diagnostic and treatment methods. However, all past experience of human development shows us that no matter how expensive and exclusive technology may be, once it enters the broader market, it quickly becomes much more accessible. Cancer has been an integral part of life for *Homo sapiens* for millennia of human culture and tens of thousands of years of evolution among early humans as well. Cancer is the evolutionary price that we pay for our multicellularity and longevity. Though it will be several decades before we are able to finally solve cancer, we are actually not far from being able to pay off this biological debt. And then, cancer will no longer be a source of horror and a curse, but rather what it should be: an interesting and scientific phenomenon, a "warped mirror" into which new generations of scientists will gaze, no longer with fear, but with relentless curiosity as they try to understand the building blocks of life.

FACT: Experts believe that, in the future, medicine should satisfy four criteria (the P4 approach)—be predictive and preventive, personalized to reflect the patient's individual features, and initiate the patient's active participation in any treatment process. The last point implies that patients should not be passive targets of medical manipulation but rather conscious and active partners working alongside their doctors.

Conclusion
MORE THAN JUST SCIENCE...

I would like to end our journey into the world of molecular oncology on a positive note. But if you have any personal motivations for picking up this book, other than purely academic curiosity, it is unlikely that you can truly share my optimism. To tell the truth, I am myself not always that convinced. If you or a loved one has been diagnosed with cancer and you find yourself frantically flipping through the pages of this book in order to wrap your head around what is happening, you are hardly comforted by knowing that one day, in the future, people will have beaten cancer or at least managed to get it under control. The disease exists now. It has gotten far less deadly than it was a hundred years ago, but it does still kill people. Prognoses vary, but there is always hope.

But what can you do, what can you think, how can you survive what is here and now? How can you find meaning in the suffering cancer causes? How can you reconcile with possibly losing a loved one, or with losing your own life, after all?

As a biomedical scientist, I am not the person to answer all of these questions, but as a person who has also experienced the death of family and friends and pondered my own mortality, I cannot help but try. I realize that I am treading on shaky ground and that any misstep might cause people even more alarm and distress, and I want to share my own experience, but I will not give my own opinion. I know a lot about the molecular mechanisms of cancer, but I certainly do not feel I know enough about human suffering to claim authority on matters of life and death. Religion offers us answers, but they are not right for everyone. However, there was a man who lived in the twentieth century who was confident that the meaning of human life persists even in the most unbearable circumstances, and that this was something we can all lean on when we feel that our spiritual strength is running on empty. At least, that is what I think as well. Of course, that is just one person's opinion, and not the absolute truth. You are certainly free to listen to other ideas or seek other ways to reconcile with yourself and with life.

The man's name was Viktor Frankl (1905–1997). He was an Austrian psychologist of Jewish descent, and a survivor of the Holocaust. Not only did he survive this ordeal without breaking, but he managed to turn the experience he gained at such a terrible price into something that would benefit humanity. Viktor Frankl founded logotherapy, a psychological approach based on finding meaning in the patient's life. Later, this method was further developed by his students. The echoes of this humanistic approach can be found in the work of many notable psychologists from the second half of the twentieth century, even those who officially belonged to completely different schools and areas.

Viktor Frankl insists that there are not and cannot be any circumstances in which human life loses all meaning. Illness and death can take a lot away from us, but they cannot deprive us of this last dignity. This is how he describes it in the most important book he wrote, *Man's Search for Meaning*:[7]

[7] Viktor Frankl, Man's Search for Meaning: An Introduction to Logotherapy. 4th ed. (Beacon Press, 1995).

"We must never forget that we may also find meaning in life even when confronted with a hopeless situation, when facing a fate that cannot be changed. For what then matters is to bear witness to the uniquely human potential at its best, which is to transform a personal tragedy into a triumph, to turn one's predicament into a human achievement. When we are no longer able to change a situation — just think of an incurable disease such as inoperable cancer — we are challenged to change ourselves."

In his book *Life Filled with Meaning: Applied Logotherapy,*[8] Frankl's student Alfried Längle gives the following example:

Mrs. B felt desperate when she was diagnosed with cancer and told that the operation would not bring much improvement. What could she do in that situation? Around the same time, she learned that her two children were planning a trip to America. She immediately saw at least one way to respond to the new circumstances — she decided not to tell her children about her illness. She knew that they would not take the only chance they had to travel if they knew about her diagnosis. With this decision, she did not allow her disease to completely control her and dictate how she should behave. She was suffering from cancer — there was nothing she could do about it now, but she felt a certain satisfaction in the fact that even in this hopeless situation, something depended on her, because she had found the answer as to why she should endure this suffering.

This story is not about patients' need to hide their disease from their loved ones — there are different families, different relationships, different circumstances. Längle reaches quite a different conclusion from this story: many people's lives show that nothing is entirely up to fate. There are things that cannot be avoided, but we also always have the power to do something, regardless of the circumstances we

[8] Alfried Längle, Sinnvoll leben: Eine praktische Anleitung der Logotherapie. 2nd ed. (Residenz Verlag, 2011) (in German).

face. However, if a person becomes fixated on the caprices of fate and tries to cancel the inevitable or change what has already taken place, they are already setting up impossible conditions, and all of their other options will gradually disappear from their field of vision. The greatest danger of fate might be that a person becomes depressed, constantly thinking of nothing but how everything could be different, happier, and better, if it were not for fate... But life does not work that way, and we cannot always select the conditions that we might like the most.

When fate strikes a blow and we realize that we are powerless to prevent it, the reason for our suffering is no longer the most important thing. That becomes secondary, because it is beyond our influence. Now, the most important thing is our decision: will we accept our suffering or try to escape fate (by denying reality or with drugs or suicide)? It is up to us to choose how we suffer and what is worth living for, whether or not we will have new relationships and values, for which, despite all the suffering, we are willing to continue living. People will suffer for the most personal things in their lives. What else, other than the very essence of a person themselves could this be? Suffering is part of the most intimate sphere of us and, therefore, it would be inappropriate to use it in order to play the hero. The most important thing here is to simply be oneself.

There are many charity organizations around the world that help cancer patients. One of them was founded recently, in 2018, by oncologist Andrey Pavlenko, who unexpectedly found himself in the role of patient when he was diagnosed with stage-three stomach cancer. As he stood on the other side, as a cancer patient rather than a physician, Pavlenko began to see all of the shortcomings of the modern Russian healthcare system from another perspective. He used his human and medical authority to draw attention to the problem, and he had barely begun to recover from serious treatment that had lasted for months, when he began to organize a foundation aimed at helping patients and improving doctors' qualifications. The story of Andrey Pavlenko once again confirms that people are stronger than their circumstances. We are capable of taking even a deadly illness and turning it into a source of inspiration, using our own suffering to help others. Fearing death and disease is only natural for mortal beings, who are aware that their time is finite. But as long as we are alive, it is in our power to resist the temptation to despair. Not everyone is able to defeat the disease, and none of us will defeat death. But it is still possible to preserve ourselves, our dignity, and our values, and leave this place undefeated.

Afterword

PATHS TO SCIENTIFIC KNOWLEDGE – THE PARABLE OF THE BLIND MEN AND THE ELEPHANT

The scientific knowledge overproduction crisis we discussed earlier gave rise to a new scientific field of study known as "systems biology." Its aim is to restore a holistic biological picture of the world at its current level of scientific development so that the life sciences do not drown in the details. In a world of narrow specializations, systems biologists try to maintain a generalized, "synthetic" view of biological phenomena and re-learn how to see the forest despite the trees.

Scientists who work in this field like to illustrate their point with the ancient Indian parable about the blind men and the elephant:

An elephant was once brought into a town. Many people wanted to see it. Among them were six blind sages. But how can you see an elephant if you are blind?

"I know," said one sage, "we will feel it with our hands."

"Good idea," said the others. "Then we will know what an elephant is like."

And so, the six sages went to "see" the elephant.

The first felt its large, flat ear. He slowly moved it back and forth. "It's a fan! An elephant is like a fan!" he exclaimed.

The second sage stood near the elephant's leg and touched it. It was round and mighty.

"Hmm... this is round and thick... An elephant is like a tree trunk!" he exclaimed.

"Neither of you are right," said the third sage. "Yes, it's round, but it's not thick, and it is very bendy! It's like a rope!" That sage had been feeling the elephant's tail.

"No, that's not it at all! An elephant is like a spear! Yes, it is round, yes, it is thin, but it doesn't bend at all!" The fourth sage was touching the elephant's tusks.

"No, no," cried the fifth, "elephants are like a high wall. Big, wide, and rough," he said, as he felt the elephant's side.

The sixth wise man was holding the elephant's trunk.

"You're all wrong," he said. "The elephant is like a snake."

"No, it's like a rope!"

"No, a snake!'

"A wall!"

"You're all wrong!"

"I'm right!"

The six blind sages began shouting at one another in a fit of rage. They went on like this for an entire day. Then another day, then a week went by, and they still could not agree. Each sage was only imagining what his own hands had felt, and only believed himself. As a result, they all thought that they were right and knew what an elephant was like. No one wanted to listen to what anyone else had to say. And so, they never knew what an elephant looked like.

As we come to the end of this book, I feel like all of those blind men at once. I tried to feel a huge phenomenon as best I could from all angles and share it with my readers. This was no easy task, but I hope I have generally managed. The artist did a good job on the elephant's tusks and tail — the question is, did I manage to draw the whole elephant? And moreover, do the details of molecular transformations and cellular reactions create a picture of cancer, not just as a disease, but with a special status of living matter? Popular mythology never stops growing — have we missed any brand-new myths?

Only you can answer that question, dear readers. I would love to hear your comments, questions, and suggestions, which you can send to international@alpina.ru, and I will certainly try to take them into account in future editions of this book.

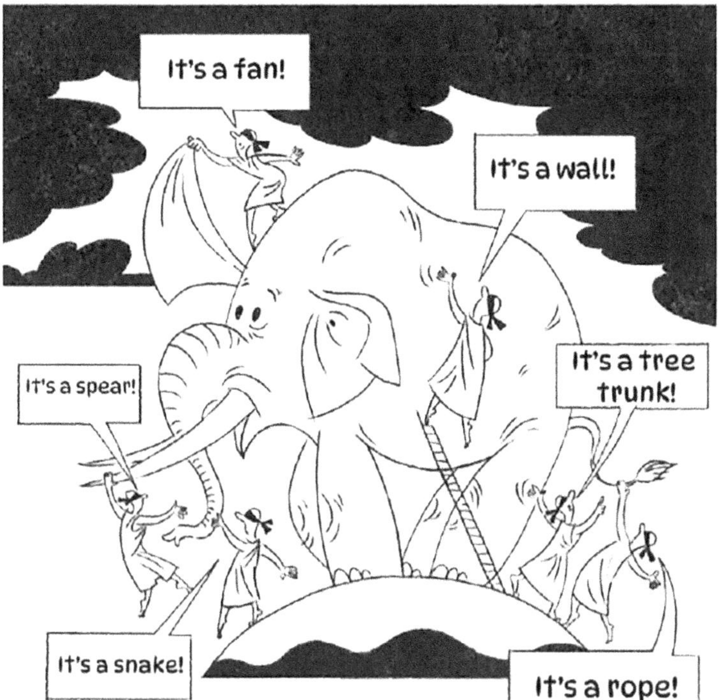
It's a fan!
It's a wall!
It's a spear!
It's a tree trunk!
It's a snake!
It's a rope!

Figure 23. The blind men and the elephant are a universal metaphor for scientific inquiry.

PS: There is an alternative tale about blindness and elephants floating around on the Internet (author unknown): "One day, six blind elephants got together in hopes of learning what humans were like. One elephant put his foot on a man and said: "People are small and flat." The other elephants also felt the man under their feet and unanimously agreed..."

Acknowledgments

I would like to thank all of my colleagues and friends whose conversations provided material for this book, and whose advice proved truly invaluable during the drafting stage and made the manuscript so much better than I had originally imagined it. Special thanks to my colleagues at the Curie Institute — Tatiana Popova, Andrey Zinoviev, Inna Kuperstein, and Ela Zueva. Their professional support and friendship were a great help as I entered the new world of molecular oncology.

The founders of the site Biomolecule, Anton Chugunov and Vera Bashmakova, inspired me to venture into popular science several years ago. It was the articles published in Biomolecule that gave shape to this book. My friends, Natalya Marchenko, Evgenia Chikalenko, and Marianna Markova were enthusiastic guinea pigs who read the first version of the book and gave me confidence that something could come out of it. My brother, Ivan Kondratov, helped write the chapter on modern approaches to drug development. I give thanks to all of them.

I would like to express my very special and endless gratitude to my parents, for bringing me into this world and teaching me to love it; my teacher Alexander Kozlenko, who introduced me to the beauty and complexity of biology; and our department head, Emmanuel Barillo, whose decision to hire me at the Curie Institute in 2014 can be considered an invisible but absolutely necessary prologue to this book.

Finally, I am immensely grateful to Pavel Podkosov, the publisher of Alpina Non-Fiction, who was enthusiastically in favor of my idea to write this book, and who then patiently waited nearly two years for me to complete it.

Bibliography

A complete list of all the literature used when writing this book would extend into the hundreds, but I doubt the practicality of such a detailed bibliography for a book on popular science.

Therefore, in compiling the final list, I leaned toward overview articles that give a more or less comprehensive view of certain areas of molecular oncology covered in this book, though there are also mentions of key experimental works cited in the text itself.

For the book in general

Alberts B., D. Bray, K. Hopkin, A.D. Johnson, A. Johnson, J. Lewis, M. Raff, K. Roberts, and P. Walter. *Essential Cell Biology*. 3rd ed. Garland Science, 2009.

Hanahan, D. and R.A. Weinberg. "Hallmarks of Cancer: The Next Generation." *Cell* 144, no. 5 (2011): 646–674.

Mukherjee S. *The Emperor of All Maladies: A Biography of Cancer*. 1st ed. Scribner, 2011.

Weinberg R.A. *The Biology of Cancer*. New York: Garland Science, 2014.

Chapter 1. MYTHS – BOTH HYSTERICAL AND HISTORICAL

Aurengo A. "Comment Marie Curie a révolutionné la médecine." *Le Figaro: Santé*, March 8, 2018.
https://sante.lefigaro.fr/article/comment-marie-curie-a-revolutionne-la-medecine

Brown J.R., and J.L. Thornton. "Percivall Pott (1714–1788) and Chimney Sweepers' Cancer of the Scrotum." *British Journal of Industrial Medicine* 14, no. 1 (1957): 68–70.

Cancer Research UK. "Cancer Survival forCommon Cancers." https://www.cancerresearchuk.org/health-professional/cancer-statistics/survival/common-cancers-compared

David A.R., and M.R. Zimmerman. "Cancer: An Old Disease, a New Disease or Something in Between?" *Nature Reviews Cancer* 10, no. 10 (2010): 728–733.

Faguet G.B. "A Brief History of Cancer: Age-Old Milestones Underlying Our Current Knowledge Database." *International Journal of Cancer* 136, no. 9 (2015): 2022–2036.

National Cancer Institute. "Online Summary of Trends in US Cancer Control Measures."
https://progressreport.cancer.gov/after/survival

Pinquart M., and P.R. Duberstein. "Depression and Cancer Mortality: A Meta-Analysis." *Psychological Medicine* 40, no. 11 (2010): 1797–1810.

Satin J. R, W. Linden, and M.J. Phillips. "Depression as a Predictor of Disease Progression and Mortality in Cancer Patients: A Meta-analysis." *Cancer* 115, no. 22 (2009): 5349–5361.

Siegel R.L., D.M. Kimberly, and J. Ahmedin. "Cancer statistics, 2017." *Cancer Journal for Clinicians* 67, no. 1 (2017): 7–30.

Skuse A. "Wombs, Worms and Wolves: Constructing Cancer in Early Modern England." *Social History of Medicine* 27, no. 4 (2014): 632–648.

Umar A., B.K. Dunn, and P. Greenwald. "Future Directions in Cancer Prevention." *Nature Reviews Cancer* 12, no. 12 (2012): 835–848.

World Health Organization. "Cancer."
https://www.who.int/news-room/fact-sheets/detail/cancer

Chapter 2. THE ENIGMA OF OUR GENOME AND MYTHS ABOUT THE NATURE OF CANCER

Ames B.N., W.E. Durston, E. Yamasaki, and F.D. Lee. "Carcinogens are Mutagens: A Simple Test System Combining Liver Homogenates for Activation and Bacteria for Detection." *Proceedings of the National Academy of Sciences* 70, no. 8 (1973): 2281–2285.

Bartel D.P., and P. J Unrau. "Constructing an RNA World." *Trends in Cell Biology* 9, no. 12 (1999): M9–M13.

Biémont C., and C. Vieira. "Genetics: Junk DNA as an Evolutionary Force." *Nature* 443, no. 7111 (2006): 521–524.

Couzin-Frankel J. "Biomedicine: The bad luck of cancer." *Science* 347, no. 6217 (2015): 12.

Petrucelli N., M.B. Daly, and T. Pal. "BRCA1- and BRCA2-Associated Hereditary Breast and Ovarian Cancer." In SourceGeneReviews® (Internet), edited by M.P. Adam, H.H. Ardinger, R.A. Pagon, S.E. Wallace, L. J.H. Bean, K. Stephens, and A. Amemiya. Seattle (WA): University of Washington, September 4, 1998, (updated December 15, 2016).

Shih C., L.C. Padhy, M. Murray, and R.A. Weinberg. "Transforming Genes of Carcinomas and Neuroblastomas Introduced into Mouse Fibroblasts." *Nature* 90, no. 5803 (1981): 261–264.

Smithers D.W. "Family Histories of 459 Patients with Cancer of the Breast." *British Journal of Cancer* 2, no. 2 (1948): 163–167.

Van Gent D.C., and R. Kanaar. "Exploiting DNA Repair Defects for Novel Cancer Therapies." *Molecular and Cellular Biology* 27, no. 14 (2016): 2145–2148.

Vogelstein B., and K.W. Kinzler. "Cancer Genes and the Pathways They Control." *Nature Medicine* 10, no. 8 (2004): 789–799.

Weinberg C.R., and D.J. Zaykin. "Is Bad Luck the Main Cause of Cancer?" *Journal of the National Cancer Institute* 107, no. 7 (2015).

Yoshida K., and Y. Miki. "Role of BRCA1 and BRCA2 as Regulators of DNA Repair, Transcription, and Cell Cycle in Response to DNA Damage." *Cancer Science* 95, no. 11 (2004): 866–871.

zur Hausen H. "Viruses in Human Cancers." *Science* 254, no. 5035 (1991): 1167–1173.

Горбань А., Хлебопрос Р. Демон Дарвина. Идея оптимальности и естественный отбор. — М.: Наука, 1988.

Киселев Л.Л., Абелев Г.И., Киселев Ф.Л. Лев Зильбер — создатель отечественной школы медицинских вирусологов // Вестник российской академии наук. 2003. Т. 73. № 7. С. 647–659.

Киселев Ф.Л., Боринская С.А. Вакцина против рака — первые успехи // Природа. 2007. № 3.

Киселев Ф.Л., Имянитов Е.Н., Киселęва Н.П., Левина Е.С. Молекулярная онкология: от вирусной теории к лечению рака. — М.: Геос, 2013.

Chapter 3. CELL DIVISION SECRETS AND MYTHS ABOUT CHEMOTHERAPY

Capdeville R., E. Buchdunger, J. Zimmermann, A. Matter "Glivec (STI571, Imatinib), a Rationally Developed, Targeted Anticancer Drug." *Nature Reviews Drug Discovery* 1, no. 7 (2002): 493–502.

Chen R., L. Shi, J. Hakenberg, B. Naughton, P. Sklar, J. Zhang, H. Zhou, et al. "Analysis of 589,306 Genomes Identifies Individuals Resilient to Severe Mendelian Childhood Diseases." *Nature Biotechnology* 34, no. 5 (2016): 531–538.

DeVita V.T. Jr, and E. Chu. "A History of Cancer Chemotherapy." *Cancer Research* 68, no. 21 (2008): 8643–8653.

Jordan V.C. "Tamoxifen as the First Targeted Long-Term Adjuvant Therapy for Breast Cancer." *Endocrine-Related Cancer* 21, no. 3 (2014): 235–246.

My Cancer Genome. "Cytotoxic Chemotherapy Mechanisms of Action." https://basicmedicalkey.com/cancer-chemotherapy-and-cytotoxic-agents/

Nowell P.C. "The Clonal Evolution of Tumor Cell Populations." *Science* 194, no. 4260 (1976): 23–28.

Vogelstein B., and K.W. Kinzler. "Cancer genes and the pathways they control." *Nature Medicine* 10, no. 8 (2004): 789–799.

Vu T., and F.X. Claret. "Trastuzumab: Updated Mechanisms of Action and Resistance in Breast Cancer." *Frontiers in Oncology* 2, no. 62 (2012), doi: 10.3389/fonc.2012.00062

White J. "Secret Superheroes." *New Scientist* 223, no. 2979 (2014): 28–29.

Зинченко В.П., Долгачева Л.П. Внутриклеточная сигнализация. — Пущино: Аналитическая микроскопия, 2003. (Электронная версия учебного пособия.)

Chapter 4. THE STORY OF HeLa AND MYTHS ABOUT DEATH AND IMMORTALITY

Abegglen L.M., A.F. Caulin, A. Chan, K. Lee, R. Robinson, M.S. Campbell, W.K. Kiso, et al. "Potential Mechanisms for Cancer Resistance in Elephants and Comparative Cellular Response to DNA Damage in Humans." *Journal of the American Medical Association* 314, no. 17 (2015): 1850–1860.

Dawson M.A., and T. Kouzarides. "Cancer Epigenetics: From Mechanism to Therapy." *Cell* 150, no. 1 (2012): 12–27.

Flynn R.L., Cox K.E., Jeitany M., Wakimoto H., Bryll A.R., Ganem N.J., Bersani F, et al. "Alternative Lengthening of Telomeres Renders Cancer Cells Hypersensitive to ATR Inhibitors." *Science* 347, no. 6219 (2015): 273–277.

Hao X., H. Luo, M. Krawczyk, W. Wei, W. Wang, J. Wang, K. Flagg, et al. "DNA Methylation Markers for Diagnosis and Prognosis of Common Cancers." *Proceedings of the National Academy of Sciences* 114, no. 28 (2017): 7414–7419.

Heyn H., and M. Esteller. "DNA Methylation Profiling in the Clinic: Applications and Challenges." *Nature Reviews Genetics* 13, no. 10 (2012): 679–692.

Jones P.A., J.P. Issa, and S. Baylin. "Targeting the Cancer Epigenome for Therapy." *Nature Reviews Genetics* 17, no. 10 (2016): 630–641.

Levine A.J., and M. Oren. "The First 30 Years of p53: Growing Ever More Complex." *Nature Reviews Cancer* 9, no. 10 (2016): 749–758.

Lin J., E. Epel, and E. Blackburn. "Telomeres and Lifestyle Factors: Roles in Cellular Aging." *Mutation Research* 730, no. 1–2 (2012): 85–89.

Nebbioso A., F.P. Tambaro, C. Dell'Aversana, and L. Altucci. "Cancer Epigenetics: Moving Forward." *PLoS Genetics* 14, no. 6 (2018): e1007362.

Ouyang L., Z. Shi., S. Zhao, F.T. Wang, T.T. Zhou, B. Liu, and J.K. Bao. "Programmed Cell Death Pathways in Cancer: A Review of Apoptosis, Autophagy and Programmed Necrosis." *Cell Proliferation* 45, no. 6 (2012): 487–498.

Reya T., S.J. Morrison, M.F. Clarke, and I.L. Weissman. "Stem Cells, Cancer, And Cancer Stem Cells." *Nature* 414, no. 6859 (2001): 105–111.

Shay J.W., and W.E. Wright. "Role of Telomeres and Telomerase in Cancer." *Seminars in Cancer Biology* 21, no. 6 (2011): 349–353.

Skloot R. *The Immortal Life of Henrietta Lacks*. Crown, 2011.

Takahashi K., and S. Yamanaka. "Induction of Pluripotent Stem Cells from Mouse Embryonic and Adult Fibroblast Cultures by Defined Factors." *Cell* 126, no. 4 (2006): 663–676.

Chapter 5. QUESTIONS ABOUT METABOLISM AND MYTHS ABOUT "EATING WELL"

Alexander J.L., I.D. Wilson, J. Teare, J.R. Marchesi, J.K. Nicholson, and J.M. Kinross. "Gut Microbiota Modulation of Chemotherapy Efficacy and Toxicity." *Nature Reviews Gastroenterology & Hepatology* 14, no. 6 (2017): 356–365.

Ambalam P., M. Raman, R.K. Purama, and M. Doble. "Probiotics, Prebiotics and Colorectal Cancer Prevention." *Best Practice & Research Clinical Gastroenterology* 30, no. 1 (2016): 119–131.

Cancer Research UK. "Diet and Cancer." https://www.cancerresearchuk.org/about-cancer/causes-of-cancer/diet-and-cancer

Gopalakrishnan V., C.N. Spencer, L. Nezi, A. Reuben, M.C. Andrews, T.V. Karpinets, P.A. Prieto, et al. "Gut Microbiome Modulates Response to Anti-PD-1 Immunotherapy in Melanoma Patients." *Science* 359, no. 6371 (2018): 97–103.

Greenwald P., C.K. Clifford, J.A. Milner, and J. Eur. "Diet and Cancer Prevention." *Cancer* 37, no. 8 (2001): 948–965.

Kelly C.R., S. Kahn, P. Kashyap, L. Laine, D. Rubin, A. Atreja, T. Moore, and G. Wu. "Update on Fecal Microbiota Transplantation 2015: Indications, Methodologies, Mechanisms, and Outlook." *Gastroenterology* 149, no. 1 (2015): 223–237.

Martinez-Outschoorn U. E., M. Peiris-Pagés, R.G. Pestell, F. Sotgia, and M.P. Lisanti. "Cancer Metabolism: A Therapeutic Perspective." *Nature Reviews Clinical Oncology* 14, no. 1 (2017): 11–31.

Ostrander G.K., K.C. Cheng, J.C. Wolf, and M.J. Wolfe. "Shark Cartilage, Cancer and the Growing Threat of Pseudoscience." *Cancer Research* 64, no. 23 (2004): 8485–8491.

Perez P.F., J. Dor., M. Leclerc, F. Levenez, J. Benyacoub, P. Serrant, I. Segura-Roggero, E.J. Schiffrin, and

A. Donnet-Hughes. "Bacterial Imprinting of the Neonatal Immune System: Lessons from Maternal Cells?" *Pediatrics* 119, no. 3 (2007): 724–732.

Schwabe R.F., and C. Jobin. "The Microbiome and Cancer." *Nature Reviews Cancer* 13, no. 11 (2013): 800–812.

Van Der Weyden M.B., R.M. Armstrong, and A.T. Gregory. "The 2005 Nobel Prize in Physiology or Medicine." *Medical Journal of Australia* 183, no. 11–12 (2005): 612–614.

Vander Heiden M.G., L.C. Cantley, and C.B. Thompson. "Understanding the Warburg Effect: The Metabolic Requirements of Cell Proliferation." *Science* 324, no. 5930 (2009): 1029–1033.

Umar A., B.K. Dunn, and P. Greenwald. "Future Directions in Cancer Prevention." *Nature Reviews Cancer* 12, no. 12 (2012): 835–848.

Chapter 6. THE TUMOR ENVIRONMENT AND MYTHS ABOUT METASTASES

Bosman F.T., and I. Stamenkovic. "Functional Structure and Composition of the Extracellular Matrix." *Journal of Pathology* 200, no. 4 (2003): 423–428.

Bussard K.M., L. Mutkus, K. Stumpf, C. Gomez-Manzano, and F.C. Marini. "Tumor-Associated Stromal Cells as Key Contributors to the Tumor Microenvironment." *Breast Cancer Research* 18, no. 1 (2016): 84.

Chaffer C.L., and R.A. Weinberg. "A Perspective on Cancer Cell Metastasis." *Science* 331, no. 6024 (2011): 1559–1564.

Cuzick J., F. Otto, J.A. Baron, P.H. Brown, J. Burn, P. Greenwald, J. Jankowski, et al. "Aspirin and Non-Steroidal Anti-Inflammatory Drugs for Cancer Prevention: An International Consensus Statement." *Lancet Oncology* 10, no. 5 (2009): 501–507.

Dvorak H.F. “Tumors: Wounds That Do Not Heal. Similarities between Tumor Stroma Generation and Wound Healing.” *New England Journal of Medicine* 315, no. 26 (1986): 1650–1659.

Folkman J. “Role of Angiogenesis in Tumor Growth and Metastasis.” *Seminars in Oncology* 29, no. 6 Suppl 16 (2002): 15–18.

Frantz C., K.M. Stewart, and V.M. Weaver. “The Extracellular Matrix at a Glance.” *Journal of Cell Science* 123, pt 24 (2010): 4195–4200.

Franzetti G.A., K. Laud-Duval, W. van der Ent, A. Brisac, M. Irondelle, S. Aubert, U. Dirksen, et al. “Cell-to-Cell Heterogeneity of EWSR1-FLI1 Activity Determines Proliferation/Migration Choices in Ewing Sarcoma Cells.” *Oncogene* 36, no. 25 (2017): 3505–3514.

Gaggioli C., S. Hooper, C. Hidalgo-Carcedo, R. Grosse, J.F. Marshall, K. Harrington, and E. Sahai. “Fibroblast-Led Collective Invasion of Carcinoma Cells with Differing Roles for RhoGTPases in Leading and Following Cells.” *Nature Cell Biology* 9, no. 12 (2007): 1392–1400.

Kalluri R. “The Biology and Function of Fibroblasts in Cancer.” *Nature Reviews Cancer* 16, no. 9 (2016): 582–598.

Kaplan R.N., R.D. Riba, S. Zacharoulis, A.H. Bramley, L. Vincent, C. Costa, D.D. MacDonald, et al. “VEGFR1-Positive Haematopoietic Bone Marrow Progenitors Initiate the Pre-Metastatic Niche.” *Nature* 438, no. 7069 (2005): 820–827.

Kessenbrock K., V. Plaks, and Z. Werb. “Matrix Metalloproteinases: Regulators of the Tumor Microenvironment.” *Cell* 141, no. 1 (2010): 52–67.

Mantovani A., P. Allavena, A. Sica, and F. Balkwill. “Cancer-Related Inflammation.” *Nature* 454, no. 7203 (2008): 436–444.

Nelson C.M., and M.J. Bissell. “Of Extracellular Matrix, Scaffolds, and Signaling: Tissue Architecture Regulates Development, Homeostasis, and Cancer.” *Annual Review of Cell and Developmental Biology* 22 (2006): 287–309.

Pachmayr E., C. Treese, and U. Stein. “Underlying Mechanisms for Distant Metastasis — Molecular Biology.” *Visceral Medicine* 33, no. 1 (2017): 11–20.

Peinado H., S. Lavotshkin, and D. Lyden. "The Secreted Factors Responsible for Pre-Metastatic Niche Formation: Old Sayings and New Thoughts." *Seminars in Cancer Biology* 21, no. 2 (2011): 139–146.

Rich R. M., P. J. Rosenfeld, C. A. Puliafito, S. R. Dubovy, J. L. Davis, H. W. Flynn, S. Gonzalez. "Short-Term Safety and Efficacy of Intravitreal Bevacizumab (Avastin) for Neovascular Age-Related Macular Degeneration." *Retina* 26, no. 5 (2006): 495–511.

Yang J., and R.A. Weinberg. "Epithelial–Mesenchymal Transition: At the Crossroads of Development and Tumor Metastasis." *Developmental Cell* 14, no. 6 (2008): 818–829.

Zimmer C. *Parasite Rex: Inside the Bizarre World of Nature's Most Dangerous Creatures*. The Free Press, 2000.

Chapter 7. THE FINER POINTS OF IDENTIFYING "THE OTHER" AND MYTHS ABOUT IMMUNITY

Blum J.S., P.A. Wearsch, and P. Cresswell. "Pathways of Antigen Processing." *Annual Review of Immunology* 31 (2013): 443–473.

Bottazzi B., E. Riboli, and A. Mantovani. "Aging, Inflammation and Cancer." *Seminars in Immunology* 40 (2018): 74–82.

June C.H., R. S. O'Connor, O.U. Kawalekar, S. Ghassemi, and M.C. Milone. "CAR T-cell immunotherapy for human cancer." *Science* 359, no. 6382 (2018): 1361–1365.

Kucerova P., and M. Cervinkova. "Spontaneous Regression of Tumour and the Role of Microbial Infection: Possibilities for Cancer Treatment." *Anticancer Drugs* 27, no. 4 (2016): 269–277.

Liu J.K. "The History of Monoclonal Antibody Development: Progress, Remaining Challenges and Future Innovations." *Annals of Medicine and Surgery (Lond)* 3, no. 4 (2014): 113–116.

Mantovani A., and A. Sica. "Macrophages, Innate Immunity and Cancer: Balance, Tolerance, and Diversity." *Current Opinion in Immunology* 22, no. 2 (2010): 231–237.

Murchison E. P. "Clonally Transmissible Cancers in Dogs and Tasmanian Devils." *Oncogene* 27 (2008): 19–30.

Murgia C., J.K. Pritchard, S.Y. Kim, A. Fassati, and R.A. Weiss. "Clonal Origin and Evolution of a Transmissible Cancer." *Cell* 26, no. 3 (2006): 477–487.

Papac R.J. "Spontaneous Regression of Cancer." *Cancer Treatment Reviews* 22, no. 6 (1996): 395–423.

Pardoll D.M. "The Blockade of Immune Checkpoints in Cancer Immunotherapy." *Nature Reviews Cancer* 12, no. 4 (2012): 252–264.

Rashidi A., and S.I. Fisher. "Spontaneous Remission of Acute Myeloid Leukemia." *Leukemia & Lymphoma* 56, no. 6 (2015): 1727–1734.

Reeves E., and E. James. "Antigen Processing and Immune Regulation in the Response to Tumours." *Immunology* 150, no. 1 (2017): 16–24.

Schreiber R.D., L.J. Old, and M.J. Smyth. "Cancer Immunoediting: Integrating Immunity's Roles in Cancer Suppression and Promotion." *Science* 331, no. 6024 (2011): 1565–1570.

Syn N.L., M. W.L. Teng, T. S.K. Mok, and R.A. Soo. "De-Novo and Acquired Resistance to Immune Checkpoint Targeting." *Lancet Oncology* 18, no. 12 (2017): e731-e741.

Vesely M.D., M.H. Kershaw, R.D. Schreiber, and M.J. Smyth. "Natural Innate and Adaptive Immunity to Cancer." *Annual Review of Immunology* 29 (2011): 235–271.

Терапевтические антитела. Спецпроект электронного журнала"Биомолекула." https://biomolecula.ru /specials /antitela

Ярилин А.А. Иммунология. — М.: ГЭОТАР-Медиа, 2010.

Chapter 8. A BRAVE NEW WORLD AND CONSPIRACY THEORIES IN ONCOLOGY

Barabasi A. L., and Z. N. Oltvai. “Network Biology: Understanding the Cell’s Functional Organization.” *Nature Reviews Genetics* 5, no. 2 (2004): 101–113.

Hood L., and S. H. Friend. “Predictive, Personalized, Preventive, Participatory (P4) Cancer Medicine.” *Nature Reviews Clinical Oncology* 8, no. 3 (2011): 184–187.

Kaitin K. I. “Deconstructing the Drug Development Process: The New Face of Innovation.” *Clinical Pharmacology & Therapeutics* 87, no. 3 (2010): 356–361.

Luo J., M. Wu, D. Gopukumar, and Y. Zhao.” Big Data Application in Biomedical Research and Health Care: A Literature Review.” *Biomedical Informatics Insights* 8 (2016): 1–10.

Masic I., M. Miokovic, and B. Muhamedagic. “Evidence Based Medicine: New Approaches and Challenges.” *Acta Informatica Medica* 16, no. 4 (2008): 219–225.

Sackett D. L., W. M. Rosenberg, J. A. Gray, R. B. Haynes, and W. S. Richardson. “Evidence Based Medicine: What It Is and What It Isn’t.” *British Medical Journal* 312, no. 7023 (1996): 71–72.

Umar A., B. K. Dunn, and P. Greenwald. “Future Directions in Cancer Prevention.” *Nature Reviews Cancer* 12, no. 12 (2012): 835–848.

US Food and Drug Administration. “The Drug Development Process.” https://www.fda.gov/forpatients/approvals/drugs/

Wikipedia. “Evidence-Based Medicine.” https://en.wikipedia.org/wiki/Evidence-based_medicine

Afterword. MORE THAN JUST SCIENCE...

Frankl, V. *Man's Search for Meaning: An Introduction to Logotherapy*. 4th ed. Beacon Press, 1995.

Längle A. *Sinnvoll leben: Eine praktische Anleitung der Logotherapie.* 2nd ed. Residenz Verlag, 2011 (in German).

Cancer. Hearing that diagnosis in a doctor's office can be terrifying. Is cancer a death sentence? Is it contagious? Will changing your diet keep you from getting cancer? If your parents had cancer, does that mean you will get it too?

Few diseases evoke such fear and are shrouded in as many myths as cancer. Author Maria Kondratova, a molecular biologist at the Curie Institute in Paris, busts the cancer myths and explains in language that anyone can understand what we know about cancers today and all the latest ways to diagnose and treat the disease. In molecular oncology — the study of cancer and ways to treat it at the molecular level — basic scientific knowledge of the genome structure and cellular regulation systems translate into medications and diagnostic methods that save thousands of lives. If you are concerned about cancer for yourself or family, this book will demystify the subject and help you make medically sound and healthy choices.

Bookshelves are full of texts for medical professionals about cancer and books for both specialists and laypeople about molecular biology. But if you are not a physician or biologist and want to understand exactly how healthy cells become malignant and the scientific basis for modern anti-cancer therapies, *Cancer: Myths, Realities, and a Blueprint for Living* is for you. In language that is easy to understand, author Maria Kondratova debunks the most common myths and misconceptions about this disease and shows how molecular oncology has advanced to successfully treat cancer — and reveals the biological mechanisms that keep all of life functioning.

"There is no more significant and, at the same time, complicated issue in biomedical science than cancer, and this book explains why this is so. But foremost, Maria Kondratova explodes outlandish but common prejudice related to the disease. This book will make readers sit up and take notice of true-life scientific challenges, and may also quite literally save people's lives."

Eugene V. Koonin, biologist and Senior Investigator at the National Center for Biotechnology Information (NCBI)

ABOUT THE AUTHOR:

Maria Kondratova has a PhD in biology. Since 2014 she has worked at the Curie Institute in Paris, France, one of the largest cancer research centers in Europe. Her current research interests are molecular oncology and immunology.

www.ingramcontent.com/pod-product-compliance
Ingram Content Group UK Ltd.
Pitfield, Milton Keynes, MK11 3LW, UK
UKHW020155290926
15471UKWH00005B/876

9 789659 314676